STANDING
IN
STRENGTH

ALSO PUBLISHED BY DAWN PUBLISHING:

Becoming Annie – The Biography of a Curious Woman
by Dawn Bates (2020)
Becoming the Champion – V1 Awareness
by Korey Carpenter (2020)
Break Down to Wake Up – Journey Beyond the Now
by Jocelyn Bellows (2020)
Slave Boy – Book 1 in the Democ-chu Series
by Nath Brye (2020)
Unlocked – Discover Your Hidden Keys
by Carmelle Crinnion (2020)

The Trilogy of Life Itself by Dawn Bates:
Friday Bridge – Becoming a Muslim, Becoming Everyone's Business
(2nd Edition, 2017)
Walaahi – A firsthand account of living through the Egyptian
Uprising and why I walked away from Islaam (2017)
Crossing The Line – A Journey of Purpose and Self-Belief (2017)

The Sacral Series by Dawn Bates:
Moana – One Woman's Journey Back to Self (2020)
Leila – A Life Renewed One Canvas at a Time (2020)
Pandora – Melting the Ice One Dive at a Time (2021)

STANDING IN STRENGTH

Inspirational Stories of Power Unleashed

CURATED BY

LAARNI MULVEY

Published by Dawn Publishing
www.dawnbates.com
The moral right of the author has been asserted.

For quantity sales or media enquiries, please contact the publisher at the website address above.

Cataloguing-in-Publication entry is available from the British Library.

ISBN: 978-1-913973-16-2 (paperback)
        978-1-913973-17-9 (ebook)

Book cover design – Miladinka Milic

This book is dedicated to the women who feel held back…feel voiceless…feel small. This is a new era of moving forward…being visible… and taking space.

I hear you, listen to you, and I see you.

"Cry in Strength, Instead of Struggle."
~ Laarni Mulvey

CONTENTS

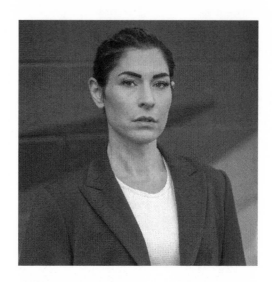

KORTNEY OLSON
USA

Kortney Olson knows what it's like to drag yourself up from the bottom. After surviving a rape, an eating disorder, depression and drug and alcohol addiction all before she was 21, Kortney knows how important it is to turn trauma, pain and despair into power, strength and confidence.

Kortney is a powerhouse speaker that will have you hooked from the very first moment. Guided by her intense passion to see women deal with their issues and take their power back, Kortney gives a no-holds barred tour into her darkest days so every woman, no matter what her story, can see there is hope on the other side. Kortney is no textbook psychologist; she knows her stuff because she's lived it. Besides being an Australian Women's arm wrestling champion, Queensland state Brazilian Jiu jitsu champion, 3-time international bodybuilding competitor, author, TV personality, Olympic lifting, kettlebell and Crossfit coach, Kortney is a self-appointed "teen whisperer", often taking time from her busy schedule to speak personally to kids struggling through puberty, bullying and the challenge of growing up in today's world. Kortney isn't just a figurehead, she gets down and dirty where it's needed most.

If you think you've seen Kortney before, it's probably because you've seen her smashing watermelons with her thighs on the Internet or TV or being described as the "woman with the world's deadliest thighs" by Stan Lee, creator of Marvel Comics; a title she holds with pride.

FOREWORD

You fight like a girl.

Don't lift too much, or you'll end up looking like your brother.

How come you can't just "tone up?"

The last thing you want is to get bulky.

God, you cry like a little bitch.

Why don't you sack up and grow a pair?

Your dad is going to need a shotgun when you get older!

Growing up, we've all heard most of these things at some point in our lives.

From adolescence, societies, religions, and cultures have programmed us to think that girls are the weaker sex. Clearly, we need protecting and have a specific rank in society. After all, it wasn't until the 1970s that a woman could get a mortgage on her own without a male cosigner in the United States. As if the mindset of being fragile wasn't enough to contend with, we've all been indoctrinated to believe that our value is equated to our exterior. Instead of chasing strength and intrinsic qualities, we've chased exterior "beauty" goals.

As a result, we have been conditioned to judge our beauty against our peers as well as other women and girls in general. This, more often than not, causes us to look at others as a threat instead of a comrade. This false paradigm of being weak and competitive for the wrong reasons has created dire statistics throughout the world in regard to girls and their mental health:

- One in five teenage girls will experience depression before they reach adulthood.
- Seven in ten girls believe that they are not good enough or don't measure up in some way, including their looks, performance in school, and relationships with friends and family members.
- Over 70 percent of girls age 14 to 17 avoid normal daily activities, such as attending school, when they feel bad about their looks.
- Eating disorders are the third most common chronic illness in young females.
- Self-harm hospital admissions have grown by over 68 percent in the last ten years, with teenage girls fifty percent more likely to self-harm than teenage boys.
- The incidence of eating disorders has doubled in the last ten years.
- Seventy-five percent of girls with low self-esteem reported engaging in negative activities like cutting, bullying, smoking, drinking, or disordered eating.

This is why we need books like *Standing in Strength* now more than ever. This book isn't just one story of strength. It's multiple stories of strength—shared by multiple different women with vastly differing perspectives. The reason why this is so important is that everyone has a different impact on people. The more variety of stories there are to identify with, the more people will be impacted.

The ability to bring a diverse group of women together with varying backgrounds, experiences, and perspectives is a reflection of what women are great at. We learn from each other in ways that are impactful and meaningful when we listen and identify with each other's stories and truths.

Growing up, I had to learn a lot of lessons the hard way. Not many people make it through drug and alcohol abuse, rape, eating disorders, depression, and addiction and come out the other side ready for world domination. But I'm not alone in having suffered. The crisis affecting the development of our society's young girls is not only terrifying but also escalating at an incredible pace.

If you knew me only from today, you'd know me as the woman with the world's deadliest thighs. If you knew me during my adolescence, you'd know that I was (in my mind) the girl with the world's fattest thighs. Seeing me today in comparison to my youth is a night and day difference. Growing up, I absolutely *loathed* my legs. I didn't have access to stories like those found in this book. Instead, I was fixated on the stories imparted on me from ads and media as a kid. Achieving a body like Kate Moss was my ultimate goal.

When I look back at my life, it startles me to think that a middle-class white girl with so much privilege and potential was still at such a high risk. I was supposed to be the first woman President of the United States of America. But instead, I got derailed by being duped into thinking methamphetamine was the answer to achieving thinness. Without the right stories, the strong women, and the right resources, I stayed off track for just over a decade before I miraculously decided to turn my mess into a message.

The transition between adolescence and adulthood is fraught with danger. Schools don't cover the issues of mental health in their curriculum, teens often can't talk to their parents, and the medical profession doesn't have the tools to help. There is literally nowhere for these young women to turn except to their peers, who are struggling to make sense of this for themselves.

So, while our societal problems grow at an alarming rate, the resources to support them have not kept pace, don't provide appropriate support, or aren't being used by girls themselves. And the resources that do exist are dealing with those young women who have spoken out or have been so damaged by their experience that society sees their need for help.

There are resources for sexually abused girls, for girls with drug problems, for girls with alcohol problems, for girls suffering the psychological impact of bullying.

But they are all dealing in cure.

A lengthy, costly, and emotionally charged process.

And only cure for those that come forward or are nominated.

The cost of dealing with just the medical side of self-harm alone is now at incredible levels. The medical intervention cost alone is estimated at $65,000,000 a year just in Australia, and in the UK it's $150,000,000 a year. In the USA, the full cost—medical, psychological, and support costs of self-harm, are a staggering $8 billion every year.

The future of care is prevention.

This is why it is so important to support work like *Standing in Strength*.

For women and girls to read stories of strength, be inspired to make change in their lives, and create a new tidal wave of women empowerment, where we can do, be, say, and lift whatever we want, is imperative.

One of the most surefire ways to give girls a fighting chance at having a stronger body image, self-esteem, and meaningful relationships with other girls is by getting them involved in athletics. Whether it be through team sports where girls learn leadership skills, confidence, and teamwork or it be through individual sports like powerlifting where they learn discipline and grit—inspiring women and girls to radically shake our current paradigm is an absolute must for the future wellbeing of our planet and fellow humankind.

If we are so busy fearing we look our worst, we can never perform at our best.

This book is our prevention.

Kortney Olson,
Founder GRRRL Clothing & Author of *Crushing It*

GRATITUDE

Mom and Dad, even though you two are no longer physically on this Earth, thank you. I would also like to thank God for giving me the strong mind and able body that gave me bravery and courage to step out of myself and share my story. I'm thankful for my husband for supporting me in this journey of being an author especially when there were many days and some nights that included "putting words down" on paper. I would also like to thank my sister for supporting me with food and being my assistant at times.

Thank you to the mentors and role models who contributed to this book. Thank you to the contributing authors. Your journeys are a valuable addition to the world to continue positive conversations to ensure upcoming generations can see there are choices and opportunities.

Thank you to my powerlifting coaches and teammates because all those conversations are cherishable moments.

Thank you to my fur babies who sat in the office day in and day out to provide their loving support when I need to walk away for a minute.

Thank you.

I Love You.

INTRODUCTION

Be strong, but not too strong so you don't look manly.

Be confident, but not too confident because it makes you look bossy.

Love yourself, but not too much. It makes you vain and arrogant.

Don't wear bright colors because wearing black makes you look thinner.

Wear your hair down because it makes you look more professional.

Two-word response.

Screw that!

How many opinions are there for women to hear?

The six women who collaborated with me in this book share the lessons they have learned from sport and where they found their strength and built their power.

They share their inner growth. Sports allows the physical and mental challenge through lessons of strength and capability. Although our experiences of strength through sport are different, we have a similarity of falling down, finding a path for growth and self-understanding.

Mine is a story of rebellion, depression, searching, then overcoming, and releasing.

I have had a power within me that has been stifled through decades of fear and cultural guilt. I had suppressed the voice of my truth so that the heat lingered in my throat like I took a bite of a ghost pepper. I could not contain the heat and the flame any longer. I wanted my voice to be heard. It was time to change the narrative of what I had been programmed to be.

For some of us, our culture programmed us. Additionally, societal expectations and the relationships and experiences we go through dictate who we become. When we finally find a stepping-stone of courage and bravery to pave our journey, the judgment, the bully, the hate, and those who feel they know better than us rear their heads. That is when our reaction will be key. Fight for who you are truly and own who you are.

Society has a perception of what women and girls can do. Women are doing more now than in past decades, but it is still a work in progress to have access to opportunity and have a united education and understanding of strong women.

I am a proud Filipino and it was time to break the mold on expectations and standards. Since I grew up not having a want to emulate anyone, I felt left to fend for myself. Searching and seeking a sense of personal identity. In my teens, though, I became a chameleon that changed my look through clothes, makeup, and interests. I people pleased every group and everyone. Underneath the unknowing and changes I was making in my self-expression, I yearned to play sports and be considered an athlete.

Being a good Filipino daughter, I complied and kept my voice a small whisper. I felt held back and unable to be myself. These feelings and thoughts took me on the roller coaster ride of waning self-confidence, self-esteem, and self-worth. As life continued, it became clear I wanted to deviate from being quiet, fragile, and submissive.

Conformity got old and boring.

I got tired of filling the usual checkboxes an Asian woman fulfills. I had enough of fitting the checkboxes. I did not fit any of the checkboxes because I wanted to make my own. I wanted to be physically strong and embrace what makes me... me. I searched for personal growth by experimenting with a lot of different activities and different people. It took learning from bad relationships with men, other people's opinions of me, and the expectations of society for me to rebel and break down walls.

In the past, I understood fitness as only to benefit me physically. In reality, fitness was a double-edged sword of wanting to be strong but not too strong because that is not how I should be seen.

A strength sport like powerlifting allowed me to see that there was a whole community out there of strong women. It took the love of sports and movement for me to connect to the right mindset. I became more loving to myself, confident, and self-reliant. Powerlifting lifted the weight of being unseen. It became the perfect balance of strength, expression, and connection. When I found powerlifting, I was able to express myself physically and grow mentally with the lessons powerlifting taught me.

It is unfortunate that society will continue to judge women using antiquated and patriarchal standards and centuries-old traditions. We are expected, as women, to follow with no hesitation.

It is time to change our role. My hope is that the next generation of women and girls see there are a variety of examples of strong women to choose from. Standing together, we can have a louder voice. We can have so much power when we go into the world together.

This collection of strength journeys are from women who found their strength through sport. Sport has given these women a different perspective and a heightened awareness of their inner power. They share what they learned about themselves in the sport they enjoy and how they got past the dreaded wall every athlete faces. This wall might have stopped them from succeeding or even trying. They talk about overcoming self-doubt, low self-esteem, and low self-confidence. These athletes, because they are all athletes in their own way, share how their successes and their failures have built their inner power. These lessons cross over from sport to life, and the women share how these lessons are useful to the upcoming generation.

This book gives you permission to love yourself and respect yourself and honor yourself. Show up as the most powerful version of you. This stronger version allows you to serve the next generation of women and be part of the collective example.

I honor these six women who have shared their inspirational stories. Their courage and their tenacity allow opening doors previously closed due to fear of being heard or using their voice. Once one door of opportunity and community opens, there's a possibility to open another door. These open doors allow others to begin their journey of knowing themselves and finding their strength.

My hope is that you find wisdom, vision, courage, and a voice through the collective stories and Stand in your Strength and Unleash the Power you have inside of you.

With love,
Laarni x

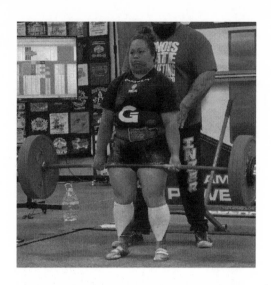

LAARNI MULVEY
USA

Filipino American women's strength advocate, author, speaker, and powerlifter, Laarni Mulvey is the founder of the Global Standing in Strength Movement.

Her 15 years working in the sports industry gave her the opportunity to learn the different perceptions of women across a multitude of sports. Learning from her personal experiences, she found an internal power that allows her to channel her voice to focus on encouraging women to harness their own unique power and strength. Using her voice to bring about global change and awareness to disrupt the narrative surrounding the perception of women, Laarni Mulvey may focus on women, and yet her message is to educate the world on the views of women and to champion them to know they are stronger than they think they are. Known as "The Power Lady," she encourages and leads women to honor themselves, and build a powerful legacy for future generations. Creator of the Tools of Strength Program, designed for use by both individuals and teams, Laarni is determined to build the connection of Strong Mind and Able Body the world over. As a women's strength advocate, Laarni is launching the Global Women's Strength Initiative to support women and girls that do not have easy access to or an understanding of strength, sports, or health and fitness. To find out more about Laarni, her work, and the Global Women's Strength Initiative, please visit https://laarnimulvey.com

CHAPTER ONE
LIFE'S A GAME OF HIDE AND SEEK

FIVE YEARS IN THE PHILIPPINES

I do not remember my childhood very much. I was born on November 24, 1976. As I write this, I will be 44, so maybe it is the suppressed memories that prevent me from remembering my childhood in detail. What I remember the most is running around being a normal kid. Enjoying childhood as much as possible in a third world country. The memories I do remember include running around with no shoes on or just some random flip flops, climbing everything, and being a mega-curious kid. Growing up in the Philippines, it was Hello Kitty and doing creative activities. Did I say Hello Kitty? Lots and lots of Hello Kitty!

Let me say this now. I love my parents and my family. I am grateful for them keeping me safe, fed, and clothed, even though shoes were a challenge. There are memories other people can rattle off left and right in their early years. Me... not so much. It is a very foggy upbringing while I was in the Philippines. What I do recall was that I was an outside kid. We had a television, but going to sit in front of it to sit and watch was something I did not purposefully do. After breakfast, I was in a rush to get outside to run around and climb trees. Even with television, I did not have the visuals of who or what I could relate to. What I was aware of was that I felt comfortable being an active kid and being creative. Athlete, athletics, sports were not words thrown around. I had no idea what sports were and had no idea what an athlete was, let alone a strong athlete that was a woman. Who would have known that deep down, I was eventually going to be considered an athlete?

One memory that supports this athlete idea was a pole attached from the brick porch post to the iron railing. Without any hesitation, I decided to reach for this bar and wanted to do a gymnast-like flip on it. Let's just say, the post won and my chin lost. Busted chin and all, I do not remember crying for a long time, but I remember the Band-Aid on my chin. Did that stop me or scare me to not do it again? Nope! I was fearless, and I was not scared to climb, reach, or do something that I did not know how to do. The rambunctious feeling in me was present. My sister and I had our own nannies, someone to take care of us other than our parents. My sister's nanny was Gloria. Gloria was awesome and so fun loving. She let me play and run around and be creative. She would join in with our playtimes, running around with us and laughing. She may have been the first person in my life that planted the seed of being an athlete in my head, but all I knew back then was that she was a whole heap of fun.

TO AMERICA I GO

One day when I was five years old, we packed up our things, hopped on a plane, and we were on a 24-hour flight to the United States. As kids we are not really told where, when, how, or anything about what is going on, you just do and go where you are told. Your parents grabbed your hand and led you where you needed to be, whether you wanted to or not. I did not know the flight was going to take us to a new opportunity. I regret so much that I never got to say goodbye to Gloria. She was possibly the first person who would have eventually shown me what sports were. I will never know.

The plane was huge, and not just because I was small, but because it was actually one of those super big planes which had two seats at each window, and I think six seats in the middle. The 24-hour-plus plane ride was an adventure. There was a slight fear and nervousness across my mother's face, and I'm not sure if it was from her first plane ride ever or the fact her English was not that great. Arriving fresh to America really was going to be an adventure, especially when realizing my mom was so nervous on the plane ride that when the flight attendant asked her if she wanted soup or salad, her answer was "yes." She thought the flight attendant asked if she wanted a "super salad!" Easy mistake to make, and one that makes me smile to this day.

There were so many people on this plane which was pulling me away from the comfort and warmth of the Philippines. I also noticed there were a lot of people who did not look like me. I knew there was going to be a big change and my curiosity was churning.

When we landed in Chicago, the vibe was already different. The hustle and bustle was faster than anything I had known before. There was a protection from my mom that made her hold my hand tighter than ever. People were all different skin colors, and no one really looked the same. It was loud and a little stinky and smelled like a musty polyester shirt that soaks up that stale body odor in the armpits. My grandparents were the ones to come get us and I was handed a pair of gym shoes. Light blue with two straps because I had yet to learn to tie laces. I remember putting them on and thinking "what the heck are these?" I may have walked around a bit like a dog that gets those winter booties and have no idea how to walk in them. "Okay Laarni, one foot in front of the other. That's it. I can do this!"

As I am looking around and soaking in my new environment, my grandma is telling my sister and I that we must speak English here and not Tagalog[1] because we were in America. As a Filipino kid, you do not question what the adults, especially an elder, says and go with it. Me, the running around rambunctious kid, was now getting programmed to become American and fit in, whatever that meant!

---

1   Tagalog—member of the Central Philippine branch of the Austronesian (Malayo-Polynesian) language family and the base for Pilipino, an official language of the Philippines, together with English. It is most closely related to Bicol and the Bisayan (Visayan) languages—Cebuano, Hiligaynon (Ilongo), and Samar. Native Tagalog speakers from the second largest linguistic and cultural group in the Philippines and number about 14 million; they are located in central Luzon and parts of Mindanao. https://www.britannica.com/topic/Tagalog-language

We lived with my grandparents on the south side of Chicago in their basement until my parents could find us a place of our own. Running around outside with no flip flops or shoes was not acceptable in my new surroundings. I had to wear shoes and couldn't go outside without permission from my aunt, who I just met and did not really know all that well. Whenever I wanted to do something, she would do this glaring squint with her eyes and would say in a tone that was a warning threat to a young kid "sige ka" in Tagalog. It was a "I said you can't go outside, see what happens if you try me" tone. Although I was told to mainly speak English since I was now in America, I still understood Tagalog.

I was an obedient kid. I listened to what my elders said and obeyed. Just like many children who listen to and respect their elders, I would still have the rebellion rising within me to push the line of what I could do or what I could get away with. At this early age, I felt the overprotectiveness and strict unspoken rules of my family deeply. The usual hierarchy of the family generations which existed in most families also existed within my own. My grandparents were the top dogs because it was their house, and as we lived with my grandparents, the rules trickled down to my dad and whomever else was living there. I am grateful for the protection though, especially given that I am an immigrant Asian girl, living in the big city of Chicago versus the gated house I lived in while in the Philippines. Those gates kept me inside the familiarity of what I knew. In the Philippines, I had the protection of similarity and seeing people who look like me. I had the protection of the iron gate and Gloria. In the United States, I didn't interact with anyone besides my sister and my parents and immediate family. Going across the street was a no-no, sitting on the porch was not allowed. Even the backyard was sometimes forbidden. I appreciate being protected as a young kid, but there was the invisible barrier that made me curious. Deep inside, I knew there was MORE. I knew I wanted MORE but the voice to ask for more was silenced because of fear.

SINK OR SWIM

In my mind, my first American school was scary and awesome at the same time. At least in my mind I figured it would be. I went to a preschool in the Philippines and it was running around and playing all day. My first bus ride to my new American school was a scary moment. I got the same uneasy and unknowing feeling in my stomach similar to getting on the two-day trek to come to the United States. This time, my mom's hand was nowhere to be held, but I was with my sister and that gave me some comfort. I got on the bus and just looked out the window, soaking up the streets and the visual of store windows. The school came closer and the bus stopped. My sister and I got off at this new unknown destination, heading off into separate directions because she was older and had to go with the older kids. Without mom there to put her hand on my back to guide me where to go, knowing I was on my own, my adventurous spirit was high, and yet laced with a mixture of excitement, curiosity, and fear. I was on my own. There were no kisses, goodbye, or statements of luck or "have a good day!"; I was on my own, left to figure it out. I had to become independent really quickly.

MY NAME HAS 2 A'S

If you did not see my name on the cover of this book, my name is Laarni. In the Philippines it's a common name. Are you trying to figure out the two a's and how to say it? It's pronounced with a pause between the two a's. La-arni.

In America, it was an alien-like name that no one has ever heard of. At my new American school, I would say my name the way it's supposed to be said. La-arni, with the pause between the two a's. My name was the first source of childhood bullying I encountered. Kids would laugh about my name because all they heard was the -arni portion of my name and they associated it with Ernie... as in Bert and Ernie from Sesame Street. So I got called Ernie, and boy did I learn to say my name with conviction. I would say "It's LA-ARNI!" They didn't care.

My name was a source of being made fun of, and I was called Ernie for a long time, even after all the corrections I gave them in how to pronounce my name. I was the kid that was called last for gym-time games, because besides having a nontraditional name, I was a tiny kid. Everyone was taller than me, and as I had Asian eyes, the kids would ask me if I could see.

I transitioned to another school in fourth grade, and with another school, it meant I had to explain how to say my name all over again. I maintained the pause in between the two a's and made sure I let people know that is how it was pronounced. I corrected teachers and other students because it is MY name! I would go on to the next grade, and the next explaining my name over and over again.

My mom's name was Rigolina. People called her Lina or Leena. I saw it spelled a few different ways on her memo pads she got from work. What was happening? Why were people not saying her name? I did not question the nickname because I figured that was how it was supposed to be and how she wanted to be addressed. She introduced herself as Lina and not by her given name. Maybe it helped my mom assimilate into American culture because she had a Filipino accent. A more "American" name possibly made her feel accepted and made people feel comfortable addressing her.

I continued the fight for my two a's. For some reason, I thought that if I left the environment of kids that made fun of me because of my name, things would be different, but I was wrong. I started hating my name because it was not an "American" name.

Throughout the years, the pronunciation of my name morphed to a more Americanized sound which made me "Hawaiian" instead of a Filipino... insert deep sigh here.

PROUD FILIPINO

I love being a Filipino and a proud immigrant. Filipinos get lumped into the Asian umbrella. There is a perception of Asians that we are expected to be meek and dainty, and to be docile and quiet. We are also expected to follow our cultural direction of who we are supposed to be. There is a silent expectation as a female Filipino to become a nurse.

On the one hand, Filipino culture has a silent matriarchal society. Mothers were really the silent boss and the driver of the family. It did not matter what her ability was, or whether she worked and/or made more money. The Filipino woman had the superpower of juggling life and the family. My mother went to business school in the Philippines to be a secretary, which is what she aspired to be. This break in the pattern of the usual Filipino woman was my example of breaking the cultural standard. She did not go to nursing school, an option offered to her and many other young women like her. She was a fun-loving woman who wanted to do what she wanted to do. When we came to the United States, she found a job at an advertising agency in downtown Chicago. I remember going down to her work and saw she was loved by everyone there. One time, she let me go into the sound booth and talk into the voice-over microphone. I heard my voice for the first time and I giggled and laughed. It brought out the idea that I had a voice. My mother worked hard, really hard, and after taking the train down to the city, she would come home and make dinner for us, do the laundry, clean the house. Although she performed the usual Filipino women duties, she had an independence that oozed out of her. BUT… she did not fulfill her independence. I feel like my mom wanted more from her life, but she settled into her life in America, became the secretary she wanted to be and took care of her family. My mother had the silent strength that I wish I would have tapped into when I was younger. By the time I wanted to talk to my mother like a mother and an adult daughter would, it was too late for me to ask her some life questions because she passed away in 2001. She died at a crucial time in my life during my early 20s.

My father was head of the household. He carried the traditional Filipino mindset with him when we moved from my grandparents' house. He was the one that took the action to make the family decisions. He was the disciplinarian. He was the one that dictated what his daughters are supposed to choose as a career. My dad followed his own independent footsteps. Instead of becoming a doctor, he became a computer analyst.

The girls of the family were expected to go to school, get straight A's, be on National Honor Society, Honor Roll, or the Dean's List at school every semester. Extracurricular activities were not allowed. I felt my dad's high expectations to succeed academically put a pressure on my shoulders. I rebelled against the standards and expectations of my culture, and of my dad. I was expected to get good grades so I could go to college to be a nurse, even though I did not want to be a nurse. I was a stereotypical "nerdy Asian." I did well academically, but academics was boring to me. I did well in school, but deep down I knew there was something missing. My five years as a child in the Philippines rooted a tree that represented an activity, creativity, and imagination. As much I wanted to continue that life, I did not have permission to live that life, simply because my dad did not allow that kind of living.

My family was not an overly emotional family. We were not "touchy feely," nor did we show too much emotion. Growing up, there were no cute drawings on the fridge, no pats on the back for getting an honor roll. Accomplishments were expected and not something extra to celebrate. I was supposed to excel in academics, it was what we did, a family expectation. Getting told "good job'" or "good work" or a hug of positive reinforcement was nonexistent. If I got an A- on my report card, the response was why is there not an A+. The word LOVE was not a predominant word heard in English or Tagalog (Mahal). Hard work was not hard enough, so work harder was planted in my mind. Self-doubt and low self-esteem were in my mindset and were getting reinforced by my cultural standards and family expectations.

LOST IN THE SUBURBS

I moved into one of the suburbs of Chicago. As I settled into my suburban life, I was exposed more and more to American life through watching television. In the Philippines, I did not watch too much television. Living with my grandparents, there was TV, but I did not get to watch much of it because all I wanted to do was play outside. I do remember watching the small black-and-white television my family had in our first apartment. It was not one of these 55" televisions. It was white, 20" dual turn knob television. It could only get the main channels and public television. Since this was in the latter half of the 80s, there was no live stream or cable. I remember watching reruns of Wonder Woman and Charlie's Angels. I had a love for Wonder Woman so much that I had the matching undershirt and undies. Anything that made me feel like her, like a hero, I wanted. I watched shows with first responders that included the police and firemen. These shows were prior to the popularity of the first responder shows of today. The women in these shows were secretaries, mothers, and wives and always had an apron on. It is interesting how the small black-and-white television was programming me to wear an apron, to be a housewife, or just take notes. I guess that is why it is called a television program: it's programming you into what is expected of you from society, government, and eventually your family. As a kid, you just think television is entertainment and something to do when you were done with your homework. American television programming is supposed to show you what was out there. The more I was seeing the more I compared myself, my culture, and my life to. More people that I felt I could aspire to be. I took these programs as real and what I should be and how I should be living. I was also seeing shows thinking my life should be like what I saw on TV. Where people hung out with their friends, riding their bikes around the neighborhood, going to parties. Families were doing things together like going to Disneyland and having dinner together. I should look like those girls on TV. I saw kids who were talking to their parents and having calm conversations. That was not my family. I barely talked to my parents. My family ate together on special occasions, but both my parents worked nine-to-five jobs, so when they came home, I did my best to not make too much noise. I learned to be quiet.

I also started comparing the shape of my body to others. When my parents would go grocery shopping, I would go straight to the magazine aisle. The fashion magazines, along with the magazines that were focused on teenage girls, would have these images of slender, perfectly made-up women and girls. I remember opening up magazines that had their height, weight, eye color, etc. on the inside of the magazine. I did not have that height, weight, or eye color. I was devastated that I was not like "them."

TRANSITION IN TURMOIL

One day at school, I reached into my backpack and there was a handwritten note that said "I am going to kick your ass." It was written in pencil. Wow. What a blow to my confidence. I did not know what I did to warrant such a threat, so I walked around the rest of the school year with a small bat in my bag. This simple piece of paper changed my mindset. I questioned everything I did. Was I too loud? Was I too friendly? Did I say something that offended? I felt like I was friendly with everyone and did not pose a threat. Was it because I did not look American? Was it because I was a stocky girl? Was it my name? I meshed in with the American world, so why was I being threatened? After this incident, I retreated into myself even more. I was scared and did not want to be seen or heard. So, together with not liking what I saw of my body in the mirror, not seeing the perfect American life I saw on television, and the repeated incidences of getting bullied, I was now in the first low point of my life.

My father was protective over his daughters like a father would be. As an adult, I appreciated my father being protective of his daughters. As a kid, it made my mind spiral into a depression. The protection made me rebel against him. I felt stifled being told I was going to be something that I did not want to be. I was not finding my own direction or allowed to develop my own view of the world. There was a fear of disappointment of not being the daughter my dad would brag about to others. I would get so angry being overprotected I would punch and kick inanimate objects, especially the couch, to get my frustrations out. I punched the door so hard that I put a hole in it. I had to choose to conform to my father and my culture versus knowing who I truly was because that made me a good daughter. I got so depressed that I became a cutter. I would cut my arms and my hands and cry, and I wanted to die. I had this desire to be me, but I had to conform to the obligation of my family. I had such a fire within me and I knew it was powerful but how was I supposed to express myself? Add on to this and the repeating thoughts of not looking like everyone else, not fitting into my environment, my almond shaped eyes, and being short and stocky, and I soon started to think that I would never fit in anywhere. My look changed a thousand times during my teenage years as I tried to figure out who I was. I was yearning to find myself and love myself.

CHASING PERFECT

When we moved to another suburb at nine years old, we started to have more things… like access to television. Growing up in the 80s, television was my only access to the outside world. Television was programming me to chase perfect. I saw the perfect family on TV. I saw myself in that perfect family I saw on TV. In my mind, the perfect family had the perfect red brick house with a pool in the backyard, and kids had perfect clothes from the name brand stores. Conversations were perfect: the kids could talk to their parents, and the parents would be so kind and understanding. The parents provided everything because their dads were doctors and lawyers, and their mothers would be home providing kids after-school snacks like apples and celery with peanut butter. The parents would fix their kids problems at the dinner table. Then it was a hug and a kiss at night.

The perception of perfection made me feel like I was not good enough because I did not have the life I saw on the TV shows. I did not look like those girls on TV. The girls I saw were tall, blonde, and looked perfect in khaki shorts with a pastel polo, with a popped-up collar and KEDZ shoes. I at least had the permanent tan. America is where we could live the perfect American dream right? Why couldn't I live the perfect American dream being a Filipino? I could not fit in that ideal because when I saw myself in the mirror, I was not tall, not skinny, not blonde, and not white. My visual of myself was not good enough. Maybe that was the reason for them bullying me. Maybe what they saw was something that they did not like. I told myself to hide and be quiet and not be seen. No voice, no action. Head down and watch your feet move forward. I wanted that perfect life, the perfect body, the perfect family. The fear of wanting perfection that I saw on television and magazines set a fear and guilt inside me. I felt that if I diverted from my family and my dad's teachings, I would not have the love and support that I saw on television.

SPORTS LOVE

My mom watched sports, so I watched sports with her. Baseball, football, basketball... any sport that was on TV, we watched. I was intrigued with movement, the cheering and yelling by the fans. It invigorated me. I was a hodgepodge of a person. I remember being in fifth grade (ten years old), I wanted to play basketball, so I played. I may not have been a starting player, but I loved the team aspect and playing a game. I also wanted to be a fashion designer, so I would draw shoes and dresses, mix colors, and draw different patterns on my sketches. This returned the feeling of creativity and activity I had in the Philippines. Basketball allowed me to run up and down the court and reminded me of the freedom I had in the Philippines. In sixth grade (11 years old), I was able to dance to Michael Jackson's Thriller as a school performance. I enjoyed movement, dancing, and creativity. These were the things that brought me joy and happiness. It muffled the feeling of the bullying from when I was younger, but it did not remove the questions of knowing who I was and who I wanted to be. I felt confident because I had friends and people liked me, or so I thought.

My mindset changed again around 12 or 13 years old. Growing up in America in the 80s, mental health was not in the forefront of importance. Was it the teenage angst that was letting me feel the mixed emotions? Whatever it was, it was fueled by American television. Seeing the perfection of these make-believe lives, I knew I was sad. I was lost. I was depressed. My awareness of depression was something I could not put my finger on. My transition from the young child mindset to the preteen mindset where I started to make decisions for myself was challenging. I was confused, seeking direction and my purpose. Maybe I was too young to know who I wanted to be and what my purpose was, but I was open to finding someone to emulate.

At 14 years old as I entered ninth grade, I still did not know who I was because I followed the wishes of my family. Going to the big school to get lost in the sea of other students, I was so nervous. School was boring, because as I have said, academics did not bring me any joy. Sitting at a desk to only be told what to know and what to believe. Independent thinking was not encouraged. I only enjoyed physical education, art class, music class, and any class that allowed me to be creative or use my hands. My new mindset brought on even more rebellion because it was my escape from conformity. My imagination was my friend. Physical activity was where I was comfortable, knowing myself, understanding myself. One weekend, my dad took my sister and I down to the park and showed us how to play tennis. Tennis became my first exposure to sports. I loved being active. My mother even started taking me to the gym with her occasionally. The gym was another place I felt like myself.

At age 15 when I was in tenth grade, I started to venture out to try new things. One time I stayed late at school because I wanted to try out for the dance team. My dad found out and came and plucked me out of the tryout. He said he did not want me shaking my butt in front of people. I was angry because I wanted to do something creative and I was feeling held back from joy. This event in my life would pull me in two different directions. One way, I wanted to do what brought me joy and happiness, and the other way, I disappointed my father and my culture. Sports and athletics were put in the background because of my obligation and cultural pressure to be small and quiet and unseen. They put Laarni in the corner.

LOSING ME

Being a teenager is always difficult. The confusion, the mental crisis and turmoil, does not help the transition from being a kid to a teenager. Throughout my teenage years, I had so many different looks. I was the clean-cut preppy kid, the emo/punk/goth kid with the flannel shirt, Doc Martens boots, dark eye makeup, to the raver-looking kid with the wide-leg jeans that were extra-long and dragged on the ground, to the girl who wore label brand clothes head to toe. I changed like a chameleon because of what I saw on TV or the people I associated with. I did not own my own identity. As a people pleaser, I became who I was to make others feel happy and to make myself fit into a group. No identity. I was still doing life on other people's terms and living by other people's standards and expectations.

During my late teens, I still did not know my identity. The one thing that was constant though, was fitness, physical activity, and movement. My mom did take me to a commercial gym occasionally as a young teenager. When I was warming up on the bike, I grabbed some magazines to pass the time. In these magazines, I saw the same women that I saw on television. They were slender and blonde, but now I started noticing their arms were really slender as well, there was not a muscle bump to be seen! Their arms were perfect without the sagging skin under the arms. Their legs were so slender that their thighs did not touch. I subconsciously compared my body with those women in those magazines. I was not close to looking like those magazine girls. I was not built like that. I had thick legs with thighs that touched all the way down to my knees, broad shoulders that prevented me from wearing button-down shirts, and a rice belly that would protrude through my pants even though I covered it with a loose shirt. Besides not knowing my identity, now I was thinking about what my body looked like. Again, I started wondering whether it was because I did not look like the magazines that I was bullied as a kid. I also started to think that my body and my Asian look was the reason boys did not like me. I did not think I was pretty or liked because I was not skinny or white.

I was slowly losing my two a's in my name. Instead of the pause between the two a's, the two a's became meshed into one syllable. It was sad because I only went along with it to make sure my name was easier for other people to pronounce. I was now losing myself and my name.

BE SMALL

In my 20s, I got into a relationship with a guy who took me to his gym. This was not a commercial gym. It was a small gym that had dumbbells that went past 55 pounds and where there were metal plates and big machines. There were posters of bodybuilders on the wall and there was a photo of the owner of the gym when he was in competition mode. In his photo, he was flexed. His muscles were huge, cut, and lean. This was the first time seeing a body like that. Even though it was on a man, I wanted those muscles. After a little bit of going there, I asked the gym owner if I could barter a membership and some guidance on bodybuilding by working at his gym. One day, I was cleaning the gym and organizing the magazines, and I opened one of those muscle magazines and I saw women that were muscular too! I knew I wanted to look muscular too. I started to train like a bodybuilder, but what I could not discipline myself to was the diet. I tried eating like a bodybuilder by having chicken and brown rice for every meal, but I could not do it because I loved food too much. I still trained, but I was realizing that I could push, pull, and lift heavier than I ever thought I could, and I enjoyed it. This gym allowed me to embrace my physical strength and be strong. It was becoming apparent that I could lift heavier than my boyfriend. People were noticing that my legs looked strong and muscular and it made me feel good about myself. I noticed that being strong and having muscle made me confident. The elated feeling of being strong and muscular swiftly deflated when my boyfriend started comparing. He compared the size of my calves to his, he made comments about the weights I was using. He did not approve that I was lifting more than him. Again, I then continued on to live by the standards or expectations of someone else. His disapproval of me made me want to become unseen and small, literally. After that comment, I tried to diet my way to small. I wanted to be thin, tall, blonde… to look American. Lift only the lighter weights to "tone."

GETTING SMALLER

Fast forward more years and another experience brought me to work on becoming a smaller version of myself. The life I had in my 30s was fun-filled with partying and drinking. I met someone that I LET in. I was alone and lonely, and when he appeared, he filled the gap of loneliness with fun, sex, and adventures. It was the distraction for me I needed at that time and I deferred to becoming what HE wanted me to be. He wanted me to be smaller. I worked out twice a day. Cardio in the morning and then weights in the afternoon. He also wanted me to be smaller mentally. I let him control me to the point I was lost in a mind that was not mine. I had no idea who I was.

"Be smaller, Laarni, it is the only way you can be accepted by him."

This experience took me on a dangerous mental ride. I was so depressed and hit a low that brought me to losing my self-worth. It was a year of uneasiness because I was going through some mental turmoil. I hated myself. I hated that I was being fake, smiling to everyone, while inside I wanted to die. I could not talk to my family about how I was feeling because according to my dad "he did not raise weak children." My family was not the best for me to talk to. My mother had already been deceased for over ten years, and I wished she was still around because I think maybe talking to her would have been better. She maybe would have understood, but even then, I would not have felt comfortable.

I remember being in my apartment after a 12-hour day of work taking care of everyone else and I was so mad, I punched the couch cushions so hard that I hit the frame of the couch and hurt my hand. I was still getting mentally tortured by questioning myself. How I was going to get through this.

What does one do when going through a depressive, physical harm state? You go to therapy, so that's what I did, and it was the best decision of my life. I went for about four months. Thank you, therapist. You helped me stay alive and become mentally stronger. I knew there was something more to me and I was going to find myself. This was my turning point. This was the point that I had enough of being someone that other people wanted me to be. It may have taken my 30 something years of life on this Earth, but I had it. I thank the jerkface that I let manipulate me. Without him, I would not have realized I am so much more than what he saw of me. I do not credit him for 100% of the pivot, but I am grateful for the lessons I learned from the experience I had through him.

THE SEED

After therapy, I felt the growth within myself. I needed to find my constant, to revisit what I enjoyed and where I felt myself my most comfortable. It was physical activity, weights, getting sweaty, getting dirty, and challenging my body. I was going back to the gym! I was going to find the thing that gave me an all-around better me. Boxing and kickboxing classes were awesome. I ran 5Ks and other distance races. I even did obstacle course races. From tennis and playing catch when I was young, to doing outdoorsy activities like frisbee, golf, and gardening.

When I was younger, I knew I was physically strong because my dad made sure I was the one mowing the lawn, cleaning the gutters, carrying the groceries, even putting down wood floors with him. As a Filipino woman I muddle the traditional perceptions of the weak, subservient Asian woman. The image of a strong woman, a strong matriarch was my mother. She was my female example of strength. She was quiet, and although she had the subservient strength, she was strong in character, physically strong too. She worked hard to additionally provide financially to the household. She cooked and cleaned and did the laundry, but she had no problem picking up heavy bags of dirt or mulch for the garden and sitting in a crouched position for hours while weeding the garden. She was the closest role model I had to what a strong woman was. She also had biceps that I admired. I was lucky to have my mother emulate the strength I was yearning for. Although I hid my strength from my mother and father, I never lost my desire to be strong. After years of hiding myself, making myself small, and not knowing my identity, I hid my strength from the world.

Moving forward, it was up to me to encourage myself to be strong. I needed to find my strength for me. I had this natural strength that I needed to find an outlet for. I was in search of a community that gave me the opportunity to be my strong self. I was in a challenging career as an athletic trainer helping others be strong and making sure they did not hurt their bodies. My career also was holding me back from using my leadership skills and my voice. As I asked to help support the women in the company, my requests were falling on the back burner. I had to suppress those feelings so hard. I wanted to voice my opinions and concerns so bad that it started burning my throat. I had to hold the fire back because I questioned if I was good enough to be in a position of leadership. The feeling of being held back was driving me insane. I knew I had to do something. I was just diagnosed with diabetes and high blood pressure, so I needed to take care of myself. I also wanted to love myself more.

STRENGTH RISING

For years, I made myself small. I made myself so small I was unseen and unheard. I had finally arrived at the point in life where I had started living the life my Filipino culture demanded of me: being quiet and meek. In my career, I let supervisors speak condescendingly towards me because I did not feel good enough, or I felt fearful about advancing in my career. Relationships with men where I took on the persona of what they wanted me to be became the norm. I let people dictate my life and what they thought I should be. It took me a few years and some therapy to build up a level of confidence to give me some baseline courage. It took me several more years to have the confidence to build my voice. I was beginning to bring my confidence and voice together. I was done making myself small for others to understand me and for me to fit in. I'd already lost my name, and I wasn't going to lose who I was ever again.

I never had a sport or a sport focus as a kid or as a teenager. I considered myself a shy, quiet kid, but when physical activity was involved, I came out of my shell, becoming happy and comfortable with myself. There were a lot of dark days trying to find my turning point, but it was those dark relationships and struggles of cultural standards which were the best lessons of my life. They pressed me to find and seek the best version of myself. I needed to know my strength would be used to better myself but also to share my strength with others. I had to stop myself from dismissing who I was.

In March 2019, I decided to honor my word to compete in the powerlifting sport. Competing was stretching my confidence and my capabilities. Though it was not bodybuilding, powerlifting included building strength physically. I made the decision to look for a coach/personal trainer. I found one that helped me build my base of knowledge and technique. In June 2019, I transitioned to a coach that focused on powerlifting and Strongman. I met three women on my first day at this gym. These women were so strong. I watched one of them squat with weights in the upper 200s and deadlift over 300 pounds.

I was in awe!

This was what I wanted to see.

Strong women.

When we actually got to sit and talk, we clicked like we had known each other for years. We believed strength in women was important and we talked about the lessons of powerlifting. How much their physical strength gave them confidence and how that strength brings a different aura in a woman. We walk with our shoulders back; we have a do not underestimate us attitude. Strong women take space and claim it for themselves. There is a voice that demands to be heard.

The powerlifting community brings a support system that is so different to anything I had ever experienced. These ladies did not just blow smoke up your butt, they gave constructive support. Even in failure, there was still cheering and clapping.

In November 2019, I did a nonsanctioned powerlifting meet. These girls that I met were alongside me the whole time. We cheered each other on, but the other women that were competing as well. Besides learning technique, I learned more about who I was. The mental shift began to happen even more and the mold that confined me was cracking more and pieces were starting to fall. I had a stronger mind and an able body.

I found more of myself through the barbell. Lifting made me feel capable of doing something that I had wanted to do for almost a decade.

I never competed in organized sports when I was younger. Deep down I had a competitive nature that was yearning to come through. There is a saying I heard about powerlifting… "The bar will tell you the truth." I believe that. The barbell keeps you wanting to get better and better, stronger and stronger. It allowed me to do something that I may never believe was possible.

For years, I lived a life that played toward the fear of disappointment. This fear that held me back from embracing and accepting my strength. My strength is my courage. My strength is my POWER. The physical change was the tip of the iceberg. Society played on my fear and made me question my body, and made me feel less than. Getting stronger reminded me that I was worthy and I possessed within me the confidence that kept me positive and moving forward. There is an unspoken expectation for Asian women to be small, do not ruffle any feathers, stay fragile. Be the smallest of small. Asian women should not be strong physically and muscles are bad. You can exercise, but being "too big" in the Asian culture is not feminine.

To those standards, I will just say… FUCK OFF. If I were to choose between being silent and small vs big, taking space, and using my voice, I will choose to get big, VERY BIG! Powerlifting has helped me defy the standard. As women are trying to get smaller, I am trying to get as big as possible, what can I say, it is that rebellious streak in me. Powerlifting demands I take up space and grow. Instead of competing with others, I compete with myself. My strength is measured by my capability and not my weight or my clothing size. The ability to gain strength through powerlifting encourages women to be bigger—and not just physically. The barbell does not care what size you are, what your nine-to-five job is, or if you have groomed yourself or not. It is between you and the bar. When your hands grasp the weight, it comes down to either you can lift the weight or you can't. Strength requires you to get stronger by confronting your familiar discomfort and accepting failures. The mold gets broken by the hammer of strength.

So many lessons I learned powerlifting extend way beyond the platform. Powerlifting helped me overcome the standards that were placed upon me and helped me be comfortable in my body. All my life, I was telling myself I needed to be smaller and thinner. I used to poke and prod and squeeze myself like a tomato to check ripeness. Now I feel myself to see how much my muscles have grown. I look in the mirror and give myself an approving head nod because I am loving my body. It looks so strong and powerlifting gave me a stronger heart. When I feel strong and confident, it helps me support others to achieve their goals. I get to share their excitement when they perform a successful lift. I get to high-five women that I know who are stronger physically than me, and there is the camaraderie with my fellow competitors.

There is nothing to prove to others in powerlifting. All I know is that it took me over 40 years to find what I exactly needed in my life to overcome my past. Lifting weights helped me get through some depression and the complacency of life. I will not make myself small anymore to fit in a mold. I own who I am now. I own my power and strength, and it feels like me. Just me, and I have written my own standard and expectation.

STEPPING THROUGH THE PUDDLE

To this day, I do not wear shoes very often. I do my best to not put on anything that I feel constricts my movement. One day, I was in my backyard and there was a puddle of water that was running off from the gutter. I walked through the puddle and then realized I forgot to grab something. Instead of turning around, I just took a few steps backwards. I contemplated this puddle. I noticed that my forward footsteps were light and had a spring in the image. I looked at the backward footsteps and they were heavy and wide like they were stuck. The puddle was the choice presented to me. The forward and backward steps were the choice. The perception of strength is not stagnant. It continues to move forward without constriction.

In powerlifting, how do you know you are moving up? Your weight totals increase! These increases do not happen overnight, they take time, discipline, and learning to make gains. Making gains takes a lot of trial and error along with lessons of failure. Having the mindset to believe in your capabilities takes time and discipline. Building self-confidence, self-esteem, and inner positivity takes lessons, takes practice, and takes knowing you are not alone.

I want to be a symbol for women to stop themselves from becoming small and shrinking. After 30+ years of standing on the sideline, I cannot stand by watching other people fighting for women. I have a voice too, and I want to use it.

There is society's perception of what it means to be a woman. Social media is still directing women in the direction of what we SHOULD be. I want women to know they have the power in their strength to be their true selves. To be authentic and committed to who they are. We are capable of being strong physically and mentally. There is no limit to what we can do.

We have the opportunity to create whatever roles or images we want to create for ourselves. There is a range of strength on the strength scale. Women can express themselves in whatever shape or form they wish to express themselves in. The definition of strength falls upon the individual. Strength does not mean you are not a woman or feminine. Strength expands the perception of womanhood. We have come a long way in the perception of only being allowed to stay at home and take care of the home and families. We have moved past the weak women that have to be seen but not be able to handle a hammer or make executive decisions. Women have evolved stronger and stronger, but it is culture that we need to educate and not feel threatened. The upcoming generations need to see that there is opportunity for them. Let us build a slew of examples that girls can have someone to look up to. Step forward through the puddle.

When you suppress the voice for so long of who you want to be, the heat starts to linger in your throat like a bite of jalapeno pepper. When you add suppressing your true self's strength for even longer, that heat increases and turns into a scorching blue flame. How long can you contain this heat, this flame? The time to release this flame is NOW. It is time we let our voices be heard. It's time to change the narrative of what we have been programmed to be. For some of us, our culture programmed us. Additionally, societal expectations and the relationships and experiences we go through dictate who we become. When we finally find a stepping-stone of courage and bravery to pave our journey, the judge, the bully, the hate, and those who feel they know better than the person who is deciding to change their path show up to hold us down. The fight to thrive begins again.

When it comes to sport, society's perception of what women and girls can do needs an update. As athletic women, we are doing more now than in past decades, but it is still a work in progress. We need to stand together to support women as strong and powerful and be an example of strength for the younger population.

It's time we listen, share, and educate our world and change **HER** story. The collection of strength journeys in this book are from women who found their strength through sport. Sport has given these women a different perspective and a heightened awareness of their inner power. They share what they learned about themselves in the sport they enjoy and how they got past the dreaded wall every athlete faces. This wall might have stopped them from succeeding or even trying. They talk about overcoming self-doubt, low self-esteem, and low self-confidence. These athletes share how their successes and their failures have built their inner power. These lessons crossover from sport to life, and they share how these lessons are useful to the upcoming generation.

REFLECTIONS

REFLECTIONS

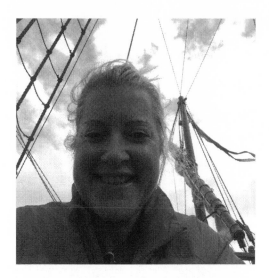

DAWN BATES
LOCATION-FREE DIGITAL NOMAD

Born in the UK, Dawn is best known for her profound wisdom, truth slaying, and high energy, not to mention a trademark giggle. As well as being an international bestselling author, author coach and strategist, and publisher, Dawn is an online entrepreneur, specializing in developing brand expansion strategies, underpinned with powerful leadership. She writes for various magazines, and when not sailing around the world on yachts, she appears on various media channels highlighting and discussing important subjects in today's society. Her first trilogy, *The Trilogy of Life Itself*, is powerful, as is her current series of nine books, *The Sacral Series*. Both compilations bring together the multifaceted aspects of the world we live in, while delivering mic-dropping inspiration, motivation, and awakening. Both bodies of work capture life around the world in all its rawness. Dawn's expertise lies in making you rethink your life, while harnessing the deepest freedom of all: your own truth. She's an authority on igniting the passions and fire deep within and shifting them from self-doubt to living life where they are free to speak and live powerfully.

To discover more about Dawn, please visit www.dawnbates.com

https://instagram.com/realdawnbates
https://facebook.com/realdawnbates
https://twitter.com/realdawnbates
Or on LinkedIn using https://linkedin.com/in/dawnbates

CHAPTER TWO
OWNING MY OVARIES

Staring down at the knife, moving my left hand to my stomach, thoughts racing through my mind, my right hand hesitated in picking it up and taking it to the excess belly fat which had taken up residence in front of me.

Cutting away the skin, which had stretched to grow with my unborn children, had its appeal, but how could I do that? To cut away the skin would be to remove the journey of pregnancy, the kisses placed on my belly by my now ex-husband, the soothing rubs and caresses I had swept over my bump and the protective cover which stopped them kicking their way out during the final stages of pregnancy.

Tears fell from my eyes, and the guilt at such a thought made my heart feel as though the heaviness which came with the guilt was crushing it into a thousand tiny pieces, until the words "Mummy, why are you crying?" came from my 4-year-old son standing behind me with a look of concern on his face which still presents itself when I think of how far I have come on this journey of loving my body.

You see, his newborn baby brother had to be born 6 weeks early by emergency c-section and I had been sick all the way through the pregnancy, so much so my exercise routine had been shelved and I had lost all energy and motivation to cook, so I had taken to eating crap. There is no other word for it. It looked like food, tasted like food, but it wasn't food. It was processed, supermarket food filled with flavorings, compounds, and chemicals, some of which are found in floor cleaners and rat poisons. High in sugar and preservatives, and I had found myself in this downward spiral of knowing it was bad for me, but the toxins and sugars in it now had me addicted. The organic, high-protein meals I had been eating for years while swimming, running, and getting my Jiu Jitsu belts seemed too far out of my reach, and I knew I had to find my way back to them, because it wasn't just my physical health that was suffering, it was my mental and emotional health. These supermarket foods were more toxic than I had realized, more than the majority of people who eat them realize.

Looking at my son, I felt as though I had stabbed myself in the heart with the knife and erased his beautiful face. How could I cut away this excess skin and belly fat, while teaching him and his brother, and my three nieces, what it meant to love themselves and the skin they're in if I was contemplating taking a knife to my own body? The simple truth was I couldn't, and being a hypocrite was not something I was prepared to be, so I told him "I am crying my darling Prince because I was just having some bad thoughts about hurting myself. Mummy misses her swimming and running, and looking like I used to, so I think today is the day I start doing them again, don't you?"

Excited about swimming, my Prince's face lit up and he responded "Yes! Let's go swimming! And you look beautiful Mummy, you just wobble a bit more like jelly, and jelly is yummy. Can we make some jelly Mummy? Please?"

How could I refuse a request like that? So, we went swimming together, I enrolled myself and his little brother into Mama and Baby swimming lessons, and my Prince into his next level of swimming. The gym was a thirty-minute walk away, and so we walked three times a week to our swimming lessons. The weight would fall off, I knew it would, I just had to be kind to myself.

The doctors had told me I wouldn't be able to do any kind of strenuous exercise for five years. In my head I had told them they didn't know me and that five years was far too bloody long. I also thought they were highly irresponsible for saying that. Who were they to tell me how long it would take me to heal my body? Who were they to tell me what my body was and wasn't capable of? Who were they to tell me anything other than the things the medical equipment they were using to detect the things I couldn't detect, when I could read medical textbooks like they had read to get them to where they were? Reading and understanding isn't rocket science, and although they went through years of medical school, and knew how to detect and look for things, I was feeling them, experiencing them, and witnessing them. I left that particular doctors' appointment with a steely determination and signed up for the local half marathon the following year. That would give me plenty of time to lose this extra 62kg I had gained.

I had doubled in weight, and to me, someone still haunted by teenage bulimia, I thought I looked awful. Disgusting in fact. So deeply brainwashed by the media and what a woman's beauty looked like, I had begun to hate my own body, the very vessel I had traveled through life in and which had been the very portal my children were conceived, developed, and been birthed by, not to mention the years of sexual pleasure and the endless achievements it had helped me gain both in business, sports, and adventures.

It was time to fall in love with my body and say, "FUCK YOU!" to the stereotypes that us women had been imprisoned by for centuries. It was time to stand in my own version of strength, love all of me, not just my mind, leading my children and nieces in the best possible way.

I told a few friends about the half marathon so they could help keep me accountable. My husband at the time was home for the next few months so he stepped up to help with the boys, but then had to go away. I was left to run the business, the household, and take care of all the duties surrounding motherhood, as well as train, so it was time to dig even deeper. If I was going to get my health and fitness back, I had to. This was not a time to use anything as an excuse. I either wanted to be healthy and see my children grow up, and become an active grandmother, or I didn't.

I had never liked looking in a mirror, so there were very few mirrors in the house, and the scales we had never got used. I never used weight as a measure, just how well my clothes fit or didn't fit, and more importantly, how far I could run or swim, or how long I could exercise for. All I knew was I was carrying far too much weight and it was impacting my lungs, livers, knees, ankles, and heart, and I hated clothing designers. I hated shopping and how it made me feel about my body, and I hated the way I looked as I walked past shop windows. They would reflect back at me this woman I didn't recognize. The woman on the outside was most definitely not the woman I felt on the inside, so she had to go. One way or another she had to go.

The half marathon training, combined with the swimming and walking, helped me lose some weight, but I was still nowhere near where I wanted to be. I had become clever at disguising how big I actually was, a size 22 in UK clothing, with many people believing I was around a size 16. The food I was eating was returning to the fresh ingredients, all homemade lunches and dinners I had been preparing before, and I felt more energized, but the weight just wasn't shifting as fast as I wanted it to. Again, the dark thoughts of having the excess cut away returned. I started looking at plastic surgery as an option.

Tummy tucks, liposuction, butt lifts, you name it, I was costing it all up. I was looking at the time it would take to generate the cash to have the surgery, how much time off work I would have following the ops, time away from the boys, where in the world I could have it all done, and what explanations I could give for my time away.

Standing in front of the mirror in the hallway, the only one I had which could give me a half decent full-length reflection, pinching several inches and rolls, I knew I would be cutting away half my body. Tears fell and I felt the fear of lying on the operating table, lights glaring, doctors chatting away to each other as if this were an everyday occurrence, which for them it was. The antiseptic smells, reminders of the c-section, and I was almost gasping for breath again with anxiety. I had always used visualizations as a tool for knowing what was to come. I would visualize the worst possible outcome, the most likely, and the absolute best outcome, and among those I would find the path I wanted to take. I looked at surgery in Brazil. It was the cheapest, and also the most tropical location so "a holiday" of sorts. Then there was the USA, where Hollywood greats had their work done, apparently. Europe and the sk:n clinic just down the road from where I lived, and on the route I had chosen as my running route. I would run past it on purpose just to make it feel like a "normal" everyday occurrence, but I knew I couldn't go through with it. For me it would be cheating, absolving me of responsibility, taking the shortcut, and avoiding the life lessons it would teach me about what I was truly capable of.

My determination to lose this weight, to become stronger and stronger the more I trained for the half marathon, which was getting closer day by day. The ex-husband was going to be back in time to be with the boys, and my friend Debbie was going to be with me, like she always was. She had been by my side every single step of the way on this journey of motherhood, and I was more married to her than I was my husband at the time. She had been the one to take me to the hospital when I couldn't breathe, stay with me, and check in on me daily. The one who took me back to the hospital when the hospital knew things were taking a turn for the worse. She rallied the troops and took care of almost everything I couldn't related to the boys... and her cooking! Masha'Allah, her cooking was amazing! Neither of us were going to be skinny eating the meals we made, but we would be healthy, and we would enjoy them, and each other's company. One of the so-called problems with food being your favorite ingredient and not working out for hours every other day is that you will never be able to maintain a lean and muscular figure, especially if you have children and sit down at work a lot. I didn't want to spend hours every day in the gym, or go without the foods I enjoyed, but I did want to love the skin I was in. Something had to give, and I had some choices to make, and quickly.

The day of the half marathon was almost upon me, and my number had arrived, so had the fundraising kit for Motor Neurone Disease, the charity I had chosen in honor of my next-door neighbor Cathy, whose body was being ravaged by the disease. Money was already rolling in, my business community and friends were getting the word out, my radio appearances had gone from business to weight loss and my personal journey, which was proving to inspire many people. I had no idea, because I didn't feel inspired. Just fat, ugly, and disappointed. Speaking about how disgusted I was with my body really triggered a lot of people, men and women alike, and it was interesting for me to discover so many men had body consciousness issues as well. How naïve we women are when it comes to the journey our male counterparts are on, even those of us who have "done the work," which at that time I had only just begun doing.

The morning of the half marathon arrived, and I knew I was not where I wanted to be physically, mentally, or emotionally in terms of loving and accepting my body, but I had said I was going to do this, and there was no way I was going to back out now. Far too many people were relying on me, watching me, and who was I to let them down? What I didn't realize at the time was it was my higher self that I wasn't prepared to let down, it was my own fears of letting others down, especially my boys who had been cheering me on and getting excited about "Mummy's medal." How could I not do this and rob them of this medal?

Walking into the crowd of runners I felt sick. Sick with anxiety, sick with envy, sick with disgust, and sick with feeling disgusted of myself. I was sick and tired of myself, and being surrounded by athletes, fit and healthy people, people who looked great in their skin, whether they felt it or not, gave me a Universal smack in the face I just was not expecting. A fire and a drive to get around this 13.2-mile course was building, and that flick of a switch I had been used to in the dojo and in my swimming kicked in. I was in the zone.

Two miles in, I stepped off a pavement and twisted my ankle. I didn't care, I would keep running, well jogging, if you could even call it that. One foot in front of the other, in "the zone of Dawn," determined, thinking of Cathy, thinking of my boys, all the people who had donated, and of the woman I wanted to become. Then I thought of each and every person who had told me I was their inspiration. I had to keep running. I had to keep moving, and then as I got to the halfway point and saw the elite athletes on their way back, I stopped. I was amazed they had got that far already and started cheering them on and clapping. I was so excited for them, and then I heard "Come on Dawn, you've got this!! Stop clapping them and keep going!!" I didn't recognize the voice, but the further I got around the course, the more I heard my name being called and people cheering me on. I heard people say, "There she is!" and the fuel that gave me, the motivation I needed to keep going, even though my hips were hurting by this point, I just had to keep putting one foot in front of the other, uphill and downhill, through the seven bloody hills of Sheffield! Why on earth had I chosen to do a half marathon in Sheffield!? Of all places! I reached the flatness of Eccy Road, almost at the halfway point, and the cheering of my name was now coming from voices I recognized. Friends were there cheering me on, cheeky cheers and verbal ass kicking were coming thick and fast, and then the words "Go Mummy!" cut through the pain and I went deeper into the zone.

I had to finish this.

I was going to finish this, for all these people, for my boys and for myself.

Heading back along Eccy Road I heard someone say, "It's harder for people like them," to which someone laughed "What to stop fucking eating?", to which the first voice responded "No, to deal with arseholes like you. You have no idea what they have been through and what led them to this point... so why aren't you running? At least they have the courage..." I didn't hear the rest of what was said, but what I had heard made me smile. Someone was fighting my corner, someone I didn't know, and again I was spurred on to just keep going.

The marker points of how far to go were my targets. One foot in front of the other, one mile marker at a time, and then I rounded the corner, and there was an ambulance with the words "High Dependency Unit" written along the side. I thought I had been "in the zone" up until that point, but in reading those words, and then seeing Debbie, and then my boys and their dad, I went up a gear, and then another. Everything and everyone around me disappeared. I was going faster, and I was now totally unaware of any of the last remaining runners I was part of. Then I saw the last half a mile sign, then the opening of the stadium we were to run into, then the track, and I knew all I had to do was run around this track and then cross the finish line.

Hearing the words "Come on Mummy! You can do it!" and seeing my boys run alongside me made me smile, want to cry, want to stop and hug them, and as I made it over the finish line, I allowed the tears I had been holding back to fall. My boys and their dad came up and hugged me, Debbie handed me some water, and I was then handed my medal. I had done it. I had completed a half marathon in three hours and thirty minutes, and all I could think of was climbing into a hot bath with a cup of tea and then sleeping until the morning.

Walking, or rather hobbling, to the car, Debbie told me she was proud of me and would catch up in the week. My husband told me he was proud of me, and put his arm around me, just as much to hold me up as much as to love on me. The boys were excited I had won a medal and my eldest was wearing it around his neck. That made every ache and pain that was now in my body and had been through my body so worth it.

I got my hot bath and cup of tea; I got my sleep the next day. I also got a very stiff body and could hardly walk the next day, but being a believer in active recovery, I kept moving. The day after the day after I was in a huge amount of pain, but I went swimming anyway to move my muscles and to take the weight of my joints. Everywhere I went, friends and strangers in the gym came up to me to congratulate me. I was back on the radio talking about what it was like, and the target I had set of £500 had been beaten by over £150.

The emotional journey and awareness of what had just happened came out in my journaling, knowing if I could complete the Sheffield half marathon, having not had the fitness or the support physically from my husband, then I could do anything. If I could put on my Adidas trainers, tracksuit bottoms and t-shirt, and wobble my way around the course with people judging me, laughing at me, and do it three and a half years earlier than the doctors said I could, well… what else was physically possible, especially as I was not a runner. My friend Lesley and I had always joked that if you saw us running you should start running too, but after this, I found myself wanting to run. I wanted to go for a run and beat my personal best. I wanted to keep the distance, but improve the time, like a race against myself. I would change routes and take steeper inclines. My fitness improved, and I felt like the weight was starting to come off, but it wasn't fast enough. I was still a size 20, just one size smaller than I had been when I had started training for the half marathon and the scales still said 62kg overweight. The lack of training, the takeouts , the pregnancy weight, the steroids I had been on in hospital, all clung to my body like a protective armor. Seeing those numbers on the scales as I hid in my bathroom, I felt like giving up, wondered what the point was, but then I saw the boys' bath toys and bath books. I smiled. They were the point. I looked in the bathroom mirror and looked deep into my eyes. The woman looking back at me I still didn't recognize. It didn't matter how much I tried to smile at her, there was no smile looking back. The cheeky sparkle had gone, and then I thought of my boys, and the sparkle made an appearance. Not a big grand entrance, but an appearance in the shadows. If they could love me, if they thought mommy was beautiful, then so could I.

I knew I was depressed. I'd had it before, and I knew I was luckier than most. The thing with depression is, though, it's a nasty thing to experience, and when it takes hold, it grips you in its grasp and doesn't want to let go. The dark thoughts of cutting away all the excess fat were still dancing in the darkness of my mind, and the light in my eyes had gone out. It didn't matter how much I put on a brave smile or how much I laughed, it didn't matter how much of a lovely person I was, I still wasn't owning it. It didn't help that my now ex-husband was spending more and more time away and seemed so distant when he came back on the weekends, but looking at myself in the mirror, I didn't blame him. I mean what man would want to stand by a woman who looked like me and declare to the world I was his wife? The judgments of myself, of what it meant to be fat, of the disgust I felt about myself, the judgments I had about others, how could I be a beautiful person on the inside if I had all of this going on inside of me? The way I would make myself wrong for being so judgmental, even though size didn't make a difference to whether I loved others or not, it was certainly making a difference to the way I loved myself and that had to stop.

I had been involved in personal development for almost a decade, but that focused on business development rather than what I was now becoming more and more aware of: The Inner Work. I knew I was the common denominator in every single thing in my life, and if I felt alone, unloved by my husband, fat and ugly, or like an imposter in business, then that all started with the way I felt about myself.

I had always kept a journal, looked back over the patterns of behavior, things I had achieved, still wanted to achieve, and recurring feelings. One night after the boys went to bed, I went into my bedroom, pulled out all the journals and started reading. What I saw was a lack of love and respect for myself going back years. Everything from my bulimia, going out taking drugs, working out to look good instead of feeling strong, pushing through goals in life and business so I could get to the next one, rather than hitting the goal and celebrating it. Reading the same things I had been writing about how I was feeling abandoned by my husband, left alone to run the businesses and raise the boys by myself, and his lack of engagement with me when he came back at weekends; his only focus was on sleeping to catch up on sleep or be with the boys. I had noted all the things he did, like let me sleep, make pancakes on Sunday for us all, but always distracted, somewhere else. I had been unhappy for a long time and living a life expected of me, rather than a life I was choosing for me, for Dawn. For the woman on the inside crying and screaming to be let out. I just couldn't hear what she was saying, who she wanted me to be, what she wanted to do, how she wanted to live her life. She was a wife, a mother, a sister to two people she didn't connect with, and in a relationship with her parents which was strained at best. I had friends, good friends, but still felt like they didn't understand me, not properly. How could they? I didn't understand myself, so no one would be able to understand me until I understood myself.

I had always been strong, mentally, physically, and emotionally. I had a deep faith in God, The Universe, Source, whatever you wanted to call it, but faith in myself was built around the concept of knowing whatever I wanted I would get eventually. How, I had no idea, but come hell or high water I would get it; unfortunately, it was more hell than high water at this present time.

Having had both the boys, and the awakening that I no longer wanted to have a business that was all about profit, it was time to close the business and make the move to Egypt. Being a mother of Palestinian Egyptian children, they had to live in at least one Arabic country to learn the language, live the life, and celebrate what it meant to be Arab, especially the food. Oh My Goddess! The food! Especially Lebanese food... the best by far in the world, very closely followed by Thai... for very different reasons. Lebanese food is what I call healthy, comfort food, whereas Thai food, well that's a taste explosion for the soul, and soul on every level.

Packing up the house was done military style; it needed to be. I was doing that by myself, while selling off and closing the business, as well as being a lone parent, a more palatable name for being a married single parent if ever there was one. Organizing the letting agent, donating clothing, furniture, and the boys showing entrepreneurial and charitable spirit by hosting garage sales was keeping me distracted from everything going on within me, and that was okay; the longer I kept busy, the more I was getting done, and the more I was achieving. That's the thing with us overachievers, we are always achieving something to make up for a lack of something else. A lack of feeling, because the feelings are too much to deal with, the wounds too deep and painful to face, so push them down and deal with them later. We haven't got time to deal with them, or time to be sick, until it all comes crashing down around us, and the crashing down around me had started with Naasir's birth, unbeknownst to me and those around me.

On the outside, everything looked great. Yeah, I was overweight, but that isn't a sign of a lack of success or happiness, especially not in the Arab world. To be overweight in many parts of the world is a sign of abundance and success because you can obviously afford food, and lots of it. A legacy from the medieval aristocracies around the world which still impacts so many cultures today. Moving day came, I'd sorted everything there was to sort out, and off we went to Egypt to live life there while we decided whether that was where we wanted to stay. Several months later the Egyptian Uprising happened and presented me with many opportunities. I got to fulfill my goal as a teacher, to help support management teams in oil companies and language centers, and to develop the leadership team of an international leadership and entrepreneurship organization. I also had time to write my first book, *Friday Bridge*, and report on what was going on in Egypt for the BBC back in the UK. Interviews from BBC World Service, Sky News, and CNN followed. I was fast becoming the British voice within Egypt that wasn't tied to a political agenda or news agency. With all this going on, there was little or no time to work out, and even if there were, the gyms and facilities that were suitable for women were incredibly expensive and would need a car to get me there; not feasible with the schedule of balancing motherhood and all these new opportunities. Again filling my time with things so I didn't have to focus on the real issue, my lack of self-love and lack of love I felt within my marriage. I knew he loved me deep down, but with everything going on around us and within our lives it was easy to explain away the lack of intimacy and future planning. We were married, of course we would be together forever. We were just dealing with some difficult external challenges which we would get through, because that's what married people did. They rode the storms together.

I took to running around the complex we lived in, and swimming in the pool while the boys had their lessons in "the club," but with the lack of money coming in from my ex-husband's efforts, I stepped up again. More students, more teaching, which meant the guilt of giving other children my time, meant I stepped up my time for them, which again meant less time for me to focus on me.

As the Uprising continued, my Arabic language and cultural understanding became more and more fluent. With that, I started to understand a lot more about the subtle nuances, and the Arabic and Islamic history I had been studying all started to make more sense to me. I predicted many things that were about to happen and would eventually happen that many of the radio presenters who interviewed me called me back on their shows and asked me how I knew what would happen. I said it was easy, you just had to look at the pattern of behaviors and events. Saying that the first time, something in me shifted internally. Saying it again, something else, and each time I said it to a different show host, it felt like something was happening inside of me, I just didn't know what. With everything I was seeing and witnessing unfold around us, I knew I didn't want to stay in Egypt, not under the regime in any way shape or form. Conversations were had, arguments followed, and before I knew it, the mother-in-law had taken her role of the nasty mother-in-law to a whole new level of existence.

Four years had passed, and although there were many great memories created, Egypt was not where I wanted to raise my children, or where I saw myself in the future. We had become parents to a beautiful fur baby, and now for me, all we needed was a second dog and our family would be complete. It was time to pack up the house, organize a home for us to return to and schooling for the boys, and yet again, I did this all by myself. Hubby was too busy reporting with the BBC and attending meetings, bringing projects to fruition. I was proud of him for the involvement he had taken in helping the people of Egypt overthrow a dictator and reporting on the real happenings, as well as mentoring others at StartUp Weekends. With everything sorted out in Egypt, and the mother-in-law throwing more spanners in the works than a spoiled raging plumber dissatisfied with his latest nightmare job, we headed back to the UK.

Seven weeks into our life back in Egypt, my father-in-law, whom I was incredibly close to, died in a car crash caused by freak rainstorm. I was alone in my grief because the husband was back in Egypt finalizing projects. Fast forward another five months, and those projects he was busy working on came to light as an affair he had been having, and our marriage was over. Eighteen years of living, working, and partying together, and he had been cheating on me the whole time. My world came crashing down around me when ten days after telling me he wanted a divorce, he jumped on a train and headed to the airport to be with his new fiancé. The boys didn't understand it any more than I did, but as their mother, I had to find the answers to as many of their questions as possible, and I had some pretty big questions to ask myself too.

With the boys at school during the days, I had time to cry, to sleep, and to walk; and walk I did. I walked my dog everywhere, to collect the boys from school, in the woods, around the village, and on weekends, the boys and I would take our dog and walk some more. I enrolled the boys back in swimming, martial arts, and football for my youngest. We would heal our pain through sports, use the training and game plans as metaphors for what was going on in our life and we would grow stronger together as a family of three, and one fur baby.

I had been setting goals and targets for myself and clients for years, now it was time to set myself some pretty big goals and targets for my health and fitness, and my business. I was the only one I could rely on now, and if I was going to achieve everything I wanted to achieve, I needed to be fighting fit for it. I registered for a two-mile open-water swim, 10km run after 10km run. The boys and I worked out together in the dojo in Mixed Martial Arts, bringing forth the years of Jiu Jitsu training I'd had back in my Oxford days, because what better analogy of getting back up again and fighting is there than a combat sport.

The sports gave us focus, the sports gave us community, and they also gave us a focus for the pain and the hurt we were feeling. I would encourage the boys to punch the pain out, kick the pain out, and use their swimming lesson as a quiet meditation time through stories and analogies, and with each one I told them, I was building my own strength; and the 65kg that was still sticking to my body like disgusting piece of chewing gum sticks to the fabric of clothing after you've been sitting on it without realizing began falling away.

I had taken the time to invest in myself, time to explore who I was now as a single mom, as a woman, as a businesswoman, and also as a human. Who was Dawn? What did I want out of life? What did I want to achieve further down the years? What kind of lifestyle did I want? How did I want to feel? And as I dug deeper and started to truly love myself, I wasn't working out to numb the pain, I was working out because I loved it. I was working out because I had finally realized that if I wanted someone to love me, I had to love myself the way I wanted to be loved, and until I loved myself, I was never going to feel deeply happy and love the skin I was in.

The more I trained the more I felt alive, the more I trained the more energy I had for the boys, my business, and for my study. The more I trained the more focus I had, and even though I had no idea about it, another curve ball was coming my way, and this one I needed to be prepared for, because it was going to take everything I had, quite literally. A new relationship seemed to be going well, and I had a nice collection of medals. Life was turning around, and I was to welcome a new fur baby into our family, and so my boys would have each other, and my fur baby would have his wife.

While in Egypt, I had written and published my first book, and one night while cooking chili, chatting away, having a rant with my dog, the idea for my second book dropped in. In seven days it was written, and seven days later it was an international bestseller on three continents. My business was growing slowly and the new curveball of being arrested and thrown in a police cell, before being wrongly accused of willful neglect and abandonment of the boys while on a road trip to Scotland, hit me like an uppercut to the rib cage followed by a roundhouse to the head. I went down and I went down hard, and here's the thing, when you have been training for your black belt, 10km runs, and 2-mile swims, you don't just build strength and stamina, you build resilience and a determination like no other and I was not going to have anyone else fuck with my family. Police Scotland had messed with the wrong Mama Bear this time. This Mama had gone ninja and she was going to bring her Mama Fire, Feminine Fire, and Sagittarius Fire to the fore and beat the bastards. And yes, I swore, I swore an oath to my boys the very first moment I held them and kissed their foreheads that I would protect them at all costs and lead them to greatness, and I was going to do just that. This would be my test, and of course, being an overachiever, I wasn't just going to pass the test, I was going to pass the test with flying colors and then I was going to do what I was great at… turning negatives into positives and writing. During this time, I knew I needed help, and that help came in the form of a cleaner, who not only cleaned for me so I could focus on building my business, but also ended up being the one who introduced my fur baby to his wife; now my family was complete—with or without a husband. I had my children and my fur babies.

With everything I was learning with the court cases and diving deep into my purpose of serving others through my business, I started writing another book, this time about the injustice, corruption, and racism of Police Scotland. Once I had finished this one, I would then have a trilogy. Looking over the books, I realized they had a theme of female empowerment and entrepreneurship running through them. Leadership, diversity, and a powerful call for awareness of self, enlightenment, and justice for all. My business was bubbling along, but I still didn't have the results I wanted, and I was feeling exhausted, but I was now getting to the guts of what my business was about. The Scotland Saga, as I called it, had taken its toll on me and had taken up a lot of my training time. I had put a lot of my focus into studying the law, criminal law, family law, and human rights law, just so I could beat the system without the hefty legal fees. I was building a business, studying, being a single mom, and although I was in a new relationship, it was turning out to be a toxic one that had brought the Scotland Saga to my door, along with feelings of rejections and being raped. My exercise had slowed down, and I knew there was a correlation somewhere, especially as the weight was starting to creep back on, which to be honest wasn't a bad thing as I had lost my boobs and my curves due to the amount of training I had been doing when I first became a single mom. I wanted my curves back, but this time I was more vigilant.

Distracted one night in one of my MMA technical and sparring training sessions, too caught up in everything that was going on in

Scotland, figuring out the new angle for my business, as well as feeling like I had let my boys down, I landed badly during a throw. The pain that shot through my shoulder made me feel faint and I had to sit out for the rest of the session. Once the initial pain was over and the next day had arrived, I realized that whatever I had done needed a specialist. The result? My MMA days were over for at least three months. My eldest son helped me dress in the morning and undress at night. We joked that his future wife would benefit. That first night of lying-in bed I cried. Why were all these things happening? Where was I out of alignment with my highest self now? I was going through everything that had been happening and I realized either things needed to change in my relationship, or it had to end; either way it could not remain as it was.

A few nights later, I was soaking in the bath while the boys enjoyed "Friday Night, Pizza and Game Night." I was listening to a podcast and within twenty minutes it had me on my knees and crying from the depths of my soul. I knew the plans I had put in place for when my youngest left school now had to be brought forward; if not, bad shit was going to keep happening. I knew if I did not honor this next level of my calling, and start living the life I wanted, then bad stuff would just keep happening. I also knew I would not be able to heal from these deep wounds in my soul, wounds that had been passed on from generation to generation, through my DNA and through lifetimes. It was time to go deeper than I had ever gone before, and to do that I had to step away from my children and hand them over to their dad for the three of them to rebuild their relationship with each other, and for him to do his part. In many cultures, it is believed that the mother raises the children for the first seven years, the father for the second, and the mentor for the third. Well, this Mama Bear had raised them for eleven and fifteen years, and now it was Papa Bear's turn. Mama was off to sail around the world on her global book tour and research her next series of books, *The Mermaid's Guides to Leadership, Culture, Women, the Environment, Food and Sailing*. A series of six books which would all go towards me getting my PhD—once

I had decided on the final thesis topic and figured out a way to do it while being location-free.

With my shoulder all strapped up, exercise was hard, especially my swimming and HIIT workouts that I was doing in the home. Walking was the only option for me, one that appealed anyway. My tailbone had made cycling painful and I had already been looking into why there was so much pain in my tailbone. Too much pressure on my shoulders from carrying the weight of wanting to heal the world. Perhaps? Maybe the result of the day I was thrown from a horse and did the very best breakfall of my life? Perhaps it was the fact my first son was born spine to spine as the doctors had suggested, whatever it was, it hurt, and some days it brought tears to my eyes just to get out of a chair.

Yoga was an on-off love affair, and everything else I could think of would cause too much movement and pain in my shoulder. I soon realized this was the Universe's way of telling me to be still, so be still I would be. I did the exercise given to me by my therapist, and over the weeks and months I started to notice an improvement. I was also almost ready to set off around the world, but again had no idea of how I was going to pay for it all with legal fees and flights to New Zealand for the boys and I, and a five-week holiday together before they returned home by themselves. "Trust the process Dawn, trust that everything is a love nudge in the right direction" kept going around and around in my head. So, trusting, relinquishing control was what I did, and within a couple of weeks I realized my beloved fur babies were about to become parents. By the time the pups arrived I had pretty much secured homes for half of them, but by the time the pups were born and four weeks old, they were all sold, and flights were booked. I had been knocked down, got back up again, and now all I had to do was win the final court case and end the relationship I was in.

I thought I only had one more court appearance, but it turned out that the guy I was seeing wasn't prepared to stand by my side all the way to the end and became a witness for the prosecutor rather than stick by my side. We had to travel back to Sheffield the day after he stepped over to the dark side, and the next night, I ended it. I couldn't be with someone who could betray me like that, but a week later, I met up with him "because I missed him" and ended up facing yet another traumatic event in my life, which meant this trip I was taking by myself was now more needed than ever; an event in my life I would go on to write about in the first book of *The Sacral Series*, a book that would drop into my consciousness in the months to come.

Back to the courtroom, I knew I would win. I had to, the boys and I were flying to New Zealand a week later. Stepping into the courtroom was like stepping into the dojo, you had to believe you would win the fight. Listening to my heartbeat as the prosecutor and my lawyer went over the case so far, and then stepping up into the witness box to deliver my statement I felt as tranquil as I did in the water. I was calm, I knew I would win, and I knew that I was eternally grateful for the strength and clarity my sports had given me. Setting the outcome in my mind had been easier because of my training. I stood strong and dominant like I had been taught to in the dojo by my Senseis: "show no weakness," and knowing that thinking someone had hurt my children is what gets me in the zone to fight the fight of my life, and here I was fighting the fight of our lives, so you bet I was going to stand strong and get in the zone of show no weakness. I walked out of the court room seven hours later with a victory. The Scotland Saga was over. I had won.

Knowing I could now I could get on with the next stage of my life, and my boys and ex-husband could work on their relationship, while I fulfilled my dream of thirty-two years of living at sea was a relief in so many ways. I had only done a two-week sail from Lowestoft to Copenhagen on the Tall Ship *Excelsior*. Sailing on yachts was something I was looking forward to, and after an incredible five weeks with my boys traveling around the North Island of New Zealand, they flew home, and I set about figuring out how to sail around the world with no boat. Again, I got my game face on and knew I would win at this, I had to. I had given up everything to do this, even handed the boys over to their dad to do this. I had told my boys I was going to sail around the world, and they would get to see the world by visiting me in lots of different countries. I had also told them I would make my business a huge success, and that this time alone would help me "catch up" on the time lost due to the Scotland Saga. When they asked me if that was a promise, I smiled because in our family we had a rule that we don't break promises. So I promised and set to work.

I knew sailing required a lot of upper body strength and also a lot of balance. I had years of swimming and martial arts under my belt, so that shouldn't be a problem. I was also not afraid of water, and I am a strong swimmer, but the stamina and focus of ocean sailing took my fitness to a whole other level. I also had an idea of how little cardio I would be able to do, but I had no idea just how sedentary sailing would be. Yes, there was a lot to do on the boats, and your core muscles and micro muscles got a workout, but unless you are racing around the world in something akin to the America's Cup, or climbing the rigging on a tall ship, then there really isn't that much of a workout.

As time passed, I had to get used to how my body shape changed, and how little the clothing companies understood women who sail. There were clothing brands who produced women's wet weather gear, but unless you were a lean and tiny woman, chances are there would be little in the way of warm clothing to keep you dry as you crossed the oceans. The only option available is men's clothing and if, like me, you have an hourglass figure with a nice pair of boobs and an arse that invites a cheeky slap from your partner, you will find it near impossible to find something that looks good. This option is not only unflattering, but also dangerous. The excess arm length, bulkiness of the torso and trousers make it cumbersome and heavy. The clothing gets caught on the rigging, the cleats, and other aspects of the yacht when moving around. Looking and feeling like the Michelin Man impacts your confidence, which is one thing you really need to be in possession of, but then again women are not supposed to be on board boats according to many sailors, unless of course they are the galley bitch, rail bait, or sailing at the captain's pleasure. Sailing is still a very sexist sport, and the men who are against women sailors are no better than the men in certain parts of the world who believe women shouldn't be driving.

With the sedentary life of sailing, and being an author combined,

I found myself relaxing and sitting a lot, and I soon began to realize that unless I got active I would soon have what I call "author's arse." I started squatting and lunging, stretching (I wouldn't call it yoga by anyone's stretch of the imagination!) and whenever the crew and I arrived in a marina, I would put on my trainers and go for a run. I would also get out my skipping rope, open up my laptop and start doing my T25 HIIT workout which I had installed on my laptop. Twenty-five minutes was just perfect, especially as sometimes it was a case of arrive on land, reprovision, and then set off again. I also started doing a lot of ocean swimming with the rips and waves providing a great amount of resistance. Investing in some Pilates bands was also one of the best things I have done. They take up such little space in my backpack and yet give me a great workout, especially around the glutes and core muscles.

As I have hit my forties, I look back over my life at all the body shapes I have had through the years due to the various sports I have done, and I consider all the amazing experiences my body has gifted me such as two wonderful children, dance floor marathons back in my raving days, camaraderie and friendships with fellow gym members, martial artists and the celebrations when new belts, medals, and personal bests have been achieved. I know I am not done with my fitness, and with menopause just around the corner, I know I am in for another shape up when it comes to how I view my body, the changing shape, and levels of fitness and strength I have. One thing is for certain though, I am determined to never allow anyone else to make me feel bad about my body, like a guy who told me at the age of eighteen that I had the worst legs he had ever seen, something that resulted in me not wanting to wear shorts or skirts for almost 20 years. I also no longer wish to have surgery, and even though as I write this I am sitting in a restaurant in Brazil, the cosmetic surgery capital of the world, I know it is no longer necessary for me to dislike my body to the extent of abusing it with countless negative thoughts, diet changes, or criticism, nor do I have any more thoughts about having parts of it cut away or boosted with silicone.

For the first time in my life, I love my body, and I listen to what she needs. If I want to work out, I will, and that varies from a long walk, a swim, an online workout, or a recorded workout. I move my body every day, and when on the move from one location to another I get to carry a 20kg backpack on my back and a rucksack weighing 10kg on my front, and in the tropics, even if it is a 10-minute walk, carrying this load is a workout and a half, and most certainly works up a sweat.

I am honored to have been asked to write a chapter in this book, *Standing in Strength*, because it is about time women started to love themselves and accept who they are at different times and phases in their lives. As women, we have the ability to grow a human being inside of us, give birth in labors which last hours, and then keep a child alive on breast milk alone for months on end. We are powerful creatures, and yet we allow society, media, and disrespectful men to make us feel crap about ourselves, which then results in us comparing and judging other women, when in fact we should be celebrating each other, encouraging and supporting each other.

It's time we owned our ovaries, ladies, and loved ourselves unconditionally, we deserve it. We've been through a lot over the centuries, and it's about time we stopped the oppression of the past and stopped oppressing and destroying each other and ourselves.

It's about time we demanded more from the clothing manufacturers, demanded equal prize winnings in sport, and demanded the social narrative be changed.

This book is one of the many steps being taken around the world to change the narrative, change the inequality in sports, and leverage the power of our voices, the strength of our messages, and lead future generations of women to love themselves on a whole new level.

Thank you Laarni for who you are, who you be, and for creating the Women's Strength Initiative. You really are The Power Lady, and to all the women reading this book, I thank you for answering the call to empower yourself, the women in your space, and the generations of women who will follow.

I will leave you with one of my favorite quotes:

Gift yourself permission, to give yourself permission to have permission, because when you do, life becomes so much more enjoyable and amazing.

With love to you all,
Dawn x

REFLECTIONS

REFLECTIONS

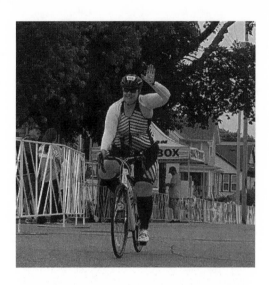

ELIZABETH SHAW
UNITED STATES

Liz Shaw is a full-time businesswoman, a part-time endurance athlete, an eating disorder survivor, a wine enthusiast, a sushi aficionado, a book hoarder, and a social media butterfly.

She found her love of endurance sports when she signed up for her first endurance event (a marathon) back in 2006 and hasn't looked back since. She has completed over 70 endurance events, including a half Ironman and a running challenge at Walt Disney World, where she ran 48.6 miles over four days. You can read more about her latest endurance endeavor at www.seelizzietri.com.

She also tends to write about the crazy antics of her life with her husband and various pets, as well as sushi and cupcakes, because a little indulgence from time to time makes everything better.

Liz's message of strength is that she wants to show that endurance athletes come in all shapes and sizes and never let someone stop you from what you want to do.

CHAPTER THREE
EVERY BODY IS BEAUTIFUL & STRONG

Remember back in grade school where there was the one kid that did not want to play dodge ball or in high school where there was one kid that would find any excuse to get out of running a mile for gym class? Well—that kid was me. Sure, I played softball and ran cross country in middle school, but I did that more to be a part of a team and the social aspect, not for the exercise. Exercising or training for something was never something I did or something that I would willingly go out of my way to do. While I heard about people getting up early on the weekends to train or workout, I was the person that would sleep in and catch up on TV shows, changing out of my pajamas just in time to go out to dinner with family or friends.

Doing an endurance event was never one of my goals or on any of my vision boards, so I shocked myself as well as friends and family when I signed up for a marathon through a charity group. For those that are wondering what an endurance event is, it is an activity (such as running) for which the person sustains a certain intensity (e.g., running speed) over a prolonged period of time. Examples of these are 5Ks,10Ks, half marathons, or marathons.

Before signing up for the marathon, the only workouts I had been doing were the elliptical trainer at the gym or a day of power shopping. Looking back—it was crazy signing up for a marathon without having even completed a 5K. The first piece of advice here—unless you have been running, I highly recommend you work your way up to the marathon. (For anyone that wants to know—yes, I did complete a 5K, 8K, and 10K before I did the marathon). I remember coming home from the informational meeting excited to share the news that I would run a marathon. While my friends and family supported my future endeavor, they didn't share the same excitement that I did, and I admit—it did take the wind out of my sails.

STRENGTH LESSON #1: DON'T LET SOMEONE ELSE'S REACTION TO YOUR NEWS CHANGE HOW YOU FEEL ABOUT YOUR GOALS OR DREAMS

During this time, I first found strength in myself to complete this goal no matter what people thought, and it lit a fire in me that I did not know I had. When I signed up for my first endurance event, I never knew I would learn so much about myself, nor that it would teach me some important lessons, nor that I would discover the strength I had deep within myself along the way.

Deciding to move forward to complete the Chicago marathon, I signed up with a local charity group. For those who are not familiar with this, the charity group will provide coaching, a training plan, group runs, and your entry into the race. In return—the runner will raise money for the chosen charity. I thought this was an excellent option for me since I was new to endurance running and needed all the help I could get, and I got the opportunity to raise money for an important cause.

I took advantage of all the training and coaching the charity group offered and attended almost all group runs. I remember when I showed up to my first group run, I realized that I was going to be one of the slower runners. I felt embarrassed and apologized multiple times for being so slow. I always felt bad because they usually waited for everyone to finish before going out for a post-run breakfast, and the last to finish was usually me. Over time, I found ways to make sure I was back in a reasonable time, so the coaching team was not kept waiting. The unfortunate part was that I started cutting my runs short—which would not help me out when it came to reaching my goal. I needed to train my body to run 26.2 miles, regardless how slow I was. Since the charity group trained for various endurance events, there were runners training for different events, and I got to meet a lot of great people, especially my people—*Back of the Packers*. I learned a little trick from them which had a big impact on my confidence within the group—start earlier so I could get my scheduled training done and finish with everyone else. To this day—I am grateful that I met them. I was close to quitting before meeting them because I felt like I just couldn't keep up with everyone else. While I appreciated all of the support the fellow fast runners and coaches provided me, I didn't feel like I was part of the group, that I belonged there. It wasn't until I met this group that I felt a sense of belonging and that I could complete this big goal I had set myself.

STRENGTH LESSON #2: DON'T APOLOGIZE FOR WHO YOU ARE, BE PROUD OF YOURSELF AND WHAT YOU CAN DO

Through meeting this group of individuals, I learned that I should not have to apologize for who I was. I was out there running the same number of miles as everyone else, and I should be proud that I was working on accomplishing this goal—no matter how long it was going to take me to complete it.

As we approached race date, the mileage increased, which also meant my anxiety around being able to finish increased. As I was starting to run more than ten miles on my long runs, I felt pretty good with the training and was becoming more and more impressed with myself. I was starting to feel like I could actually do this! I was completing all the long runs and was learning what I needed to do (and not do) during the race.

Our last long run and post-run picnic was hosted on the Chicago lakefront, with all the other charity teams. For those who are not from the Chicagoland area, running on the lakefront means you are running along Lake Michigan, and depending where you are on the lakefront, you can see the iconic skyline with all the skyscrapers or some of our famous buildings. This is one of my favorite places to run, and while I was excited to be running along the lakefront, I started to feel intimidated and nervous. Remember that **Strength Lesson #2 "Don't apologize for who you are, be proud of yourself and what you can do"** I shared with you? I forgot all about it once I was surrounded by all these runners that looked like marathon runners. You know the type—you see them on covers of magazines or on TV at the major sporting events. Even my tried and true trick of starting early did not help me. Once I got out there, people who started after me passed me, and I felt defeated. I not only felt like I would not finish the training run, I also felt like I had no chance to finish a marathon. I started getting in my head and thinking of all the people that donated to my run and letting them down if I did not finish the race. I stopped enjoying the run, stopped enjoying my super awesome playlist I created especially for that run. I stopped enjoying the comments and conversations with fellow runners, and I stopped enjoying the view on the lakefront. I just stopped and had a full-on panic attack. Thankfully one of the coaches saw me and helped me slow my breathing down, and talked me through the panic attack. At that moment, I didn't realize I was having a panic attack. I just assumed something was wrong with me. I did the walk of shame back to the starting point where my car was and ended up going home before anyone else finished and had a chance to see me leaving defeated. I was embarrassed that I didn't finish the run and didn't want to celebrate because I felt there wasn't anything for me to celebrate. I let the fear of the unknown take away from what could have been an enjoyable run and celebration of completing the long run with my fellow teammates. The following weekend I had another go, this time by myself, and I completed the long run. I wasn't doing it to prove anything to anyone other than myself; I was doing it to prove to myself that I could do it, that I was ready for the marathon, and proving both to myself was a huge step forward for me.

STRENGTH LESSON #3: DON'T LET YOUR FEAR STOP YOU FROM DOING SOMETHING YOU KNOW YOU CAN DO

Fear took away something that I knew that I could do. Fear made up stories in my head that made me believe that I couldn't do it. Choosing to silence the stories in your head that fear creates and choosing to listen to your heart and the confidence within yourself instead means you can achieve whatever you set your mind to.

I am proud to say that on October 22nd, 2006, I completed my first marathon in 7 hours 13 minutes. It was one of my proudest moments at that time because I finished a goal that I had set for myself, and I could call myself a marathoner. I was proud because I finished this goal and I did not fear what other people thought of me, nor did I allow it to stop me, which was a first for me.

After completing my first marathon and sitting on my couch watching all the bad TV my brain could handle for a couple of months, a friend of mine reached out and said she wanted to do a triathlon. Since I am willing to try anything once (well—except for skydiving), I decided to join her and a group of women to do a triathlon. I freely admit, once I decided I wanted to do this, I had to Google to understand what a triathlon was and what it entailed. For those that are not familiar with triathlons, an athlete will first swim, then transition to the bike, and after the bike will then transition to a run.

There are different distances for triathlons:

Sprint: .46-mile swim, 12.4-mile bike, and 3.1-mile run

Intermediate/Olympic: .93-mile swim, 24.8-mile bike and 6.2-mile run

Half Ironman: 1.2-mile swim, 56-mile bike, and 13.1-mile run

Ironman: 2.4-mile swim, 112-mile bike, and 26.2-mile run

While the training mentality is similar to training for a marathon, it is different because you have to train for the swim, the bike ride, and a run, and train them together, which are called brick workouts. A brick work is where you complete a swim and bike workout or a bike and run workout back-to-back. I didn't know what I was doing, but I do know I was having fun. I was training and building a bond with some amazing women using a plan that one of the women in the group had created. We didn't care about how fast we were; we just cared that we could complete the distances. While I enjoyed the charity group's training for my marathon, I only trained with them on the weekends and never really formed a bond with anyone like I did with these women. Everyone was there to train with each other, to support each other, and to celebrate with each other. It was never about the speed; it was about having fun. I never realized how much I needed support until I started training with these women.

STRENGTH LESSON #4: LET PEOPLE HELP YOU OUT—YOU NEVER KNOW WHEN YOU NEED SUPPORT

These women taught me that I could ask for help when I need it. Each one of them was there for me in one way or another whether it was to go for a run (no matter how slow I was), or to go swimming and help me with my stroke, or just have someone to talk to about any concerns or questions I had.

As we got closer to the event, I needed to find proper gear to wear for the race; I needed something I could wear for the swim and easily transition to the bike. While doing some more research (what would I have done if I didn't have the internet?), I knew I could not be like some of the pro athletes that just wore a swimsuit (hello!? Chafing!), but I could rock a tri suit like I saw other pro athletes wearing. I started my search for a tri suit that would fit me, which was not an easy feat. Oh— did I forget to tell you? I don't look like your typical lean, muscular endurance athlete, and I race in a division called Athena.

The Athena competitive divisions are based on weight minimums outlined in the USA Triathlon Competitive Rules. Athletes competing in the Athena division must be a minimum of 165 pounds. When I started triathlons back in 2007, tri suits for Athenas were hard to find, and if you did find something, it usually costs more than a pair of designer shoes. I never ended up finding a tri suit that didn't cost me an arm and a leg, so I ended up wearing a pair of men's tri shorts over my swimsuit. I believe that if you cannot make something work, then improvise, so it does work. I may not have looked cute in a tri suit like some of my fellow athletes, but I found something that worked so I could focus on the race. Thankfully, times have changed, and as more and more Athena athletes have entered the world of triathlon, athletic companies have taken notice. They have extended their size selections, and companies such as RSport (www.rsportlife.com) have started specializing in Athena apparel. Thanks to all these companies that offer Athena apparel, I now have a large selection of tri suits and shorts to choose from for my races.

STRENGTH LESSON #5: DON'T LET SOMEONE TELL YOU DON'T BELONG, BECAUSE YOU DO!

Being an Athena triathlete, and the challenges of finding the right suit, I learned that just because I did not look like an Olympic athlete, nor had the triathlon apparel of an Olympic athlete, I still belonged. I trained just as hard and had the same passion and fire as anyone else in the world of triathlons.

Race day was here, and I was ready to take on my first triathlon. The triathlon that my friend had selected was a women's-only triathlon, so the energy from all the women and the stories that they shared was amazing. The other great part about the women's-only triathlon is it wasn't as competitive as some other triathlons, making it an excellent race for a first-timer. I kept telling my friends and family that I wanted to finish the race in three hours. Since I didn't know what the race would be like for me, I decided not to pressure myself with unrealistic goals.

Little did I know that it would not take me three hours to finish the sprint triathlon—I completed my first sprint triathlon in 2 hours and 42 minutes! I remember crossing the finish line with the biggest smile on my face. I had accomplished another endurance goal that I set for myself. I was ecstatic that I'd finished, and I didn't even care about the time. The feeling when you cross the finish is something I cannot even explain. The closest example I can give is it is like every holiday you can imagine all rolled up together.

STRENGTH LESSON #6: JUST HAVE FUN! FIND THE JOY IN WHAT YOU DO AND CELEBRATE IT

After I finished my first triathlon, I was hooked. I wanted to do more, and I realized I had found my new love. I love the challenges triathlons provide as I am training for three different sports. I love that triathlons give me the ability to challenge and push myself outside of my comfort zone. I invested in upgrading my equipment; I invested in training; I invested in me. In some ways, I felt liberated when I was training and racing, like I had a purpose or had found meaning in my life. While I continued to do triathlons with my group of friends for a couple more years, I decided that I wanted to try the longer distance triathlons. I completed multiple Olympic triathlons, consisting of a .93-mile swim, a 24.85-mile bike ride, and a 6.2-mile run. Over time, our small group of triathletes dwindled to none, but I continued running races and triathlons on my own. While I was completely fine training and racing on my own, I realized that I missed the camaraderie of training buddies. On one particularly cold morning, while I was running a local race, I ended up meeting someone who was also a fellow triathlete and they told me about a training group in our area. I got excited because it was just what I was looking for at the right time.

After doing some internet stalking, I found the courage to reach out and attend an informational meeting. Following the meeting, I decided to join the group and attend indoor training sessions at the local bike shop. When I joined the group, I found out that some of the triathletes were about to start training for a half Ironman. Someone had suggested that I join them and start training for the half Ironman. I balked at that idea because there was no way I could finish a half Ironman. But then I started thinking, "But what if I could?" After thinking it over some more, I decided to take the leap and start training for my first half Ironman. I was now taking on the biggest race I had ever done—a 1.2-mile swim, a 56-mile bike, and a 13.1-mile run.

It was so great to find a group to train with, as well as an indoor cycle studio to train in during the winter months. For anyone that has cycled indoors, you know it can be boring at times, so it was fun to train with other folks, chat, and watch movies. Training for my first half Ironman progressed and I felt good, until I started having foot pain. I shook it off as training pains, but when they continued, it was recommended that I get an X-ray on my foot because there was a concern it was something worse. After multiple X-rays and MRIs, it was determined that I had stress fractures in all of my metatarsals in my right foot. This obviously was not the news I wanted to hear so early on in the training for my first half Ironman. While it was caught early on in my training, by the time I would have recovered, I would not have enough time to train safely and complete the half Ironman.

STRENGTH LESSON #7: LISTEN AND TAKE CARE OF YOUR BODY—YOU ONLY HAVE ONE

Through this lesson, I learned that it is so important to listen to your body. If you are going to do something that puts an unusual amount of stress on the various parts of your body, you need to listen to and acknowledge every ache and pain you feel. You also have to honor your body and take rest days when needed to give your body a chance to rest and heal. Ignoring the pain or not taking rest days because you feel you need to train more will only result in an injury, or several injuries.

After the diagnosis of the stress fractures and getting a stylish new boot, I decided to continue training, well, swimming and biking, with some strength conditioning thrown in, as well as spending time focusing on getting better.

Since I now had the goal in my head, I was determined to complete a half Ironman, even though it wasn't until I'd met this training group that I realized I wanted to do a half Ironman. Sure, I had talked about doing some of the longer races but never really put a plan into motion. During this period, someone came to me and told me that "If I wanted to get faster, I would need to lose weight." I was shocked at first because my weight was never a factor or a concern of anyone, but now it was? This unfortunate trigger took me down a common downward spiral that is more common than we know with endurance athletes; I developed an eating disorder. I had become obsessed with how many calories I put into my body and how many calories I burned, not caring about the nutrient-dense food I needed to eat to be able to complete such a high level of training. I went to extreme measures to manage how many calories I was consuming. I developed a toxic relationship with food where I classified food as "good" or "bad" and would only eat food that was on my prescribed diet. I associated my feelings and emotions with food. If I ate something that was not on my prescribed diet or I decided to have a piece of pizza, I felt guilt and shame.

Before I take you down this journey, I should preface that this person's comments weren't the reason I turned to such extreme measures to lose weight. I have always had a tumultuous relationship with food and with my body. I have always been overweight since I was young and was always on some kind of diet in hopes to lose weight, to look like and fit in with the other girls. The girls that could shop at any store and not have to worry if they have a selection of plus size clothes for you to choose from. Someone once asked me, "When did you start not liking your body?" and the sad part is it started when I was in high school when I was teased for my size—all I know is that for the longest time, I always wanted to fit in and look like the other girls. Through every significant milestone in my life, I was on some sort of diet to lose weight, to fit into a prom dress, to look good for graduation, to fit into a wedding dress; you get the drill. I used to joke that I was a professional dieter, I knew about almost every diet that was out there. I was on another "journey to get healthy" when I received a flyer from the charity group and thought training for a marathon would help me with this journey. For anyone that is wondering, you most likely will not lose weight when training for a marathon.

I was introduced to a diet that was used by many other endurance athletes, so I figured it had to be good, right? I decided to do this diet because I wanted to fit in with this new group, and I thought that required losing weight. I was connected with another coach (and spending more money) who wrote out a meal plan for me each week that I had to follow if I wanted to lose weight. Since I was not new to dieting, the program was not hard to follow. The hardest part was eating completely different foods as my family and friends, which brought up feelings of being separated from them all. I didn't want to go out for dinner or drinks because of an irrational fear that I could not follow what was on my meal plan if I went out. I became cranky and irritable because I was cooking two different dinners almost every night, and all because of the diet and wanting to fit in. I spent a lot of money on a diet geared towards athletes and saw success with it and got positive reinforcement from people telling me how great I looked. However, deep down, I never felt so miserable in my life.

Over time I was losing weight; however, I became obsessed with the numbers on the scale, the size label in my pants, and as I started categorizing food as "good" or "bad," I was developing fears of eating particular food items. When I didn't see results on the scale or I had a bad training day, I thought it was because I overate on my weekly "cheat" day prescribed for me, or the nutrition coach gave me too much to eat. I then found myself restricting more and more because I was so determined to succeed with this plan. Remember **Strength Lesson #3 (Don't let your fear stop you from doing something you know you can do)**—this was the one time this lesson worked against me. I was so afraid that I would fail at another diet that I was going to do whatever it took to be successful.

Around this time, someone I trained with noticed some of the unhealthy eating habits that I was practicing and mentioned to me that she had a name of a nutritionist that could help me out. While I thanked her, I did tell them that I was already working with someone on my diet. This person indicated that this nutritionist worked with individuals that had an eating disorder. I couldn't believe what I was hearing! How could I have an eating disorder? I was losing weight and following the plan. I was successful! I was so determined to prove this person wrong that I continued with the diet and was determined to work harder than I had ever. My wake-up call for me that made me realize that I needed to get help was when I decided to do a race with my friends, and even to this date, I have no recollection of the details of the race. I had been up sick the night before but was determined to do the race, a simple 5K, with my friends. We did the race, and once it was over, I started feeling sick and skipped out on the post-race lunch to go home and rest. I ended up going home and sleeping for almost 12 hours, which caused a lot of concerns for friends and family because I was not answering any calls or messages. I had wondered if I had caused this simply by not eating or not eating enough. After this race, I realized that I needed help and reached out to the nutritionist that was recommended to me.

STRENGTH LESSON #8: LOVE YOUR BODY FOR ALL THE AMAZING THINGS IT CAN DO

If there is one lesson to take away from my story, it is that you need to love your body. I have thankfully learned over time through the help of my nutritionist and therapist to love my body and to take care of it. I am also lucky because I have a great support system in my family and friends to help me through this journey. Looking back now as I write my story, I didn't love my body, I abused it. I didn't nourish it with the food it needed after hard workouts, and I punished it when it was just trying to survive.

Now that I had acknowledged I had an eating disorder and was starting on a recovery journey, I still wanted to work on that goal of a half Ironman. I had this goal in my head and was determined to complete it. I realized that I could not go back to the environment I was in because I did not want anything to jeopardize my recovery. Acknowledging that I was capable of training for this race on my own but not knowing how I needed to train, I ended up hiring a triathlon coach to work with me on a one-on-one basis versus the group plan I had previously been using. While my coach was remote, I was able to talk to her throughout my weekly training and had monthly phone calls with her. I don't know if she ever knew this, but her words of encouragement and support meant the world to me. Since I was in recovery, I felt vulnerable or concerned that some of the weight I had gained was going to jeopardize my goal of completing the half Ironman. Her words of encouragement kept reminding me of **Strength Lesson #2 (Don't apologize for who you are, be proud of yourself and what you can do)**.

The training was going well for me, and as I was getting closer to the race, I felt like I could really do this. I had the support of my coach and my nutritionist, my therapist, and my friends and family now believed I could do this. I decided to go up early for race weekend on my own as I wanted to fully embrace this experience. While my husband is my biggest supporter, the idea of walking around a race expo is not his cup of tea. The whole experience of a race put on by Ironman was something that I had not experienced before. At first, I was very intimidated to be there because I almost forgot about **Strength Lesson #5 (Don't let someone tell you don't belong because you do!)**, but once I checked in and people wished me "good luck" and "have a great race," I knew I was meant to be there, I was a triathlete, I belonged there.

Race morning arrived, and I admit I had nerves that I had never felt before on race day. As I was checked in by the officials and entered into the transition area, I got choked up and started crying. I am not sure if it was because of nerves, or after everything I had been through, I was finally at the starting line of the half Ironman. It wasn't until I found my spot and gathered myself when I heard the race officials' announcement that the swim was canceled. No! I was here for the full half Ironman experience, which included the swim! Due to the water temperature and the athletes' safety, the swim was canceled, which meant we were going to be doing a rolling start for the bike. A rolling start is where they will let a couple of athletes go every minute or so to start the bike. Now I need to tell you about this bike start—it is not like your ordinary bike start. It is at the bottom of a huge hill, and you have a very little runway to get a good start to get up the hill. Since I am not the best at hill-climbing on the bike, and while I trained for this hill, I decided to run up the hill with my bike in my bike shoes, which is not an easy feat. I figured I'd rather lose a couple of minutes on my bike by running up the hill with my bike versus falling off my bike or, worse, running into another athlete when climbing up this hill. I let any fear I had about people laughing at me because I wasn't riding up the hill go, and everyone was so supportive as I ran up the hill with my bike. I had people cheer me on, wish me good luck, and even high-five me.

Once I was at the top of the hill, I was ready to take on the 56-mile bike ride. While the ride was a challenge, I was grateful for the training I had done as well as for seeing my tribe supporting and cheering me on. I was ecstatic to have finished the ride and had a huge smile on my face as I rode down that huge hill to the transition area.

After the bike, I only had 13.1-miles to go, and then I could say I did a half Ironman, okay technically 69.1, but close enough. The great part about the race is that the run was two loops so that I could see my tribe multiple times, but you also got to see all the runners on the course, regardless of which loop they were on. I used to be so intimidated by the faster triathletes and felt their words of encouragement were something they just said to a slower athlete, but it wasn't until this race that I realized they meant it. We were all out there together doing the same miles and facing the same challenges together. Seeing everyone on the run and the support of the race crew pumped me up for the run. When I hit the second loop, I knew I would finish this race because I had made the time cutoffs for the run. Even when I was on my second loop and one of the last people on the course (I was getting my money's worth!), the energy was still there. The race crew, fellow back of the packers, and my awesome tribe were all cheering me on. That moment when I saw the finishing chute for the race is a memory that I will cherish for a lifetime. Through all the challenges I had experienced, I had finished my first half Ironman. Before you even ask, yes, I cried like a baby when I crossed that finish line, and NO! there is no shame in that.

While I relish and celebrate my first half Ironman experience,

I know I will go back and do another half Ironman to get the full experience of the swim, bike, run.

STRENGTH LESSON #9: NEVER DOUBT YOUR ABILITY TO REACH A GOAL

In training for the half Ironman as well as all the endurance races, I realized that the more races I trained for that doubt I had in myself went away. In racing, I found confidence in myself to finish a race or a goal I set for myself.

Throughout this chapter, you have read about the joy of seeing my tribe, and I would be remiss if I did not talk about my amazing tribe whom I met during my triathlon journey.

Now this tribe which I speak of, only one person in my tribe does triathlons, and she is located in another state, while the rest are runners. I met one of my tribe members at our local gym, she was the outgoing person that had this energy that you just wanted to be a part of. Over time we became friends, and she introduced me to other people that also became part of my tribe. Since they were runners, I now had people to run with in the evenings during the week or on the weekend. Some of my fondest memories during my training were meeting friends for a run in the evening during the week and having dinner afterward laughing at crazy things, such as the number of calories in a cookie butter shake from Steak and Shake and the number of burpees I would do if I had one. My tribe and I would continue to train and race at various races throughout the United States. There is one particular race that I do want to share that my friends and I did, and that was the Dopey Challenge. You probably wonder what the heck the Dopey Challenge is, and before you ask, yes, it is a Disney race. This challenge happens on marathon weekend at Disney World, and basically, you are completing all the races on marathon weekend. That would entail doing 3.1 miles, 6.2 miles, 13.1 miles, and then 26.2 miles over four days, totaling 48.6 miles. Some of my tribe members had done it before, and someone in our tribe decided they wanted to do the race, and because

I am someone that will try anything once, I signed up. I jokingly tell people the only reason I signed up for the race was FOMO (fear of missing out). I mean, if my tribe was going to be having fun (HA!) running at Disney, I wanted to be there too. Plus, there is the bling; you walk away from the race with six medals.

Physically, Dopey was hard, but mentally it was harder. You have this idea in your head you just finished a race, and you could celebrate, but no. With Dopey, you had to get up again the next morning to race again. I have said multiple times to friends and family that I would do a full Ironman before doing Dopey again. The biggest challenge with Dopey that I had is that while I was still in recovery from my eating disorder, there were times where I'd let the negative self-talk I had developed creep into my mind. Thoughts such as "I was too big to run that many races," or "You are too slow to finish," or "You look fat in your running outfit." Unfortunately, I let this dark cloud hang over me while I was doing something fun and spending time with my tribe. While I should have been able to celebrate this amazing accomplishment, I was sad and mad that I was so slow and questioned whether I could really call myself a finisher with such a slow pace. I also almost lost a significant friendship over this because I was too embarrassed to share how I felt and wouldn't let her support me when I needed it. If Dopey has taught me anything, it is to trust your tribe and let them be there for you through the good times and the bad.

STRENGTH LESSON #10: FIND YOUR TRIBE—THEY WILL SUPPORT YOU THROUGH THE GOOD TIMES AND THE BAD

I used to be one of those people who held everything in and didn't talk to people about what I was feeling or look for support from someone. I saw it as being a burden, and the last thing I wanted to do was to be a burden on anyone, especially this group of friends, my tribe. It was through this strength lesson that I learned that this is what they are there for, to support you, to listen to you, to help you get through the hard times and celebrate the good times. Looking back, I don't know where I would be without my tribe.

After fourteen years and over seventy endurance races, it still feels weird to say that I am an endurance athlete. There wasn't any one magical moment in my journey when I felt like an endurance athlete; it just naturally became part of my life and part of who I am.

So, where does that leave me today? I have been on a journey of healing for the past couple of years and feel ready to take on new challenges, share my message with others, and just have fun! Remember **Strength Lesson #6 (Just have fun! Find the joy in what you do and celebrate it**)? That became part of my mantra as I continued to recover from my eating disorder.

My mantra is, "I train and race for fun!" At some point in my training, it stopped being fun for me. It became a chore, like something I had to do, not something I wanted to do. I am happy to say that I found my joy again with triathlons. Training and racing is something that I look forward to doing. I get to celebrate the awesome workouts, and learn from the not so awesome ones. Plus, it is really fun to go out for pancakes with your friends after a great run or having sushi as a pre-race meal, and not worry about if it is part of your meal plan.

To recap, here are the ten strength lessons I have provided to you:

Strength Lesson #1:
Don't let someone else's reaction to your news change how you feel about your goals or dreams

Strength Lesson #2:
Don't apologize for who you are, be proud of yourself and what you can do

Strength Lesson #3:
Don't let your fear stop you from doing something you know you can do

Strength Lesson #4:
Let people help you out, you never know when you need support

Strength Lesson #5:
Don't let someone tell you don't belong, because you do!

Strength Lesson #6:
Just have fun! Find the joy in what you do and celebrate it

Strength Lesson #7:
Listen and take care of your body—you only have one body

Strength Lesson #8:
Love your body for all the amazing things it can do

Strength Lesson #9:
Never doubt your ability to reach a goal

Strength Lesson #10:
Find your tribe! They will support you through the good times and the bad

What I hope you take away from the story I have shared with you is that you can do whatever you want to do, just don't let fear get to you, or allow someone to tell you you can't. Don't let yourself believe you don't belong, because you do! Having the desire and drive to do something means you do belong. Go out there and meet people that want or do the things you want to do. Find your tribe because they will be your biggest supporters. Want to ride a unicycle, then do it! Want to hike Mount Kilimanjaro, then train and listen to your body as you train and go out there and do it! Want to spend the day power shopping the latest sales, go have fun doing it and don't let someone ruin your joy. While I wished someone had shared these lessons with me when I started my journey into endurance sports, I don't regret the time I spent learning these lessons on my own. I believe these lessons have made me stronger and helped me evolve into the woman and athlete that I am today. Not to toot my own horn or anything, but I do think I am kind of a badass, and I want you to feel the same way about yourself, whatever you choose to do. Go out there and have fun, celebrate your body, and believe in yourself, because I believe in you, and you should too.

With positivity and love,
Liz!

REFLECTIONS

REFLECTIONS

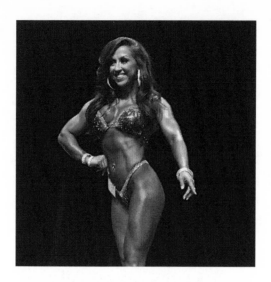

HEIDI DEHNEL
UNITED STATES

Heidi Dehnel is a former Hula dancer who originates from the Big Island of Hawaii where she received her bachelor's degree in Kinesiology at the University of Hawaii of Hilo. She, along with her husband Deven, owns Core Strength & Performance Gym in Huntsville, Alabama, where she pursues her passion as a strength coach, powerlifting meet director, and national officiate.

Understanding the impact strength training had on her own life, Heidi always hoped to grow the sport of powerlifting among the women in North Alabama. Over time, she developed "Core Barbell" an offshoot of the gym that focuses on powerlifting and that has grown to over 15 athletes, of which 85% are women.

Since launching her podcast *The Future Is Female Powerlifting* in 2018, Heidi has been able to reach more women who might be fearful towards taking the next step in strength training through powerful storytelling and intimate conversation.

Core Barbell website: https://core256.com/online-powerlifting/

Gym's FB: https://www.facebook.com/Coresandp

Gym's IG: https://www.instagram.com/coresandp/

The podcast IG: https://www.instagram.com/stories/ futureisfemalepowerlifting/2493902409806493177/

The podcast website: http://thefutureisfemalepowerlifting.com/

CHAPTER FOUR

SHE STOOD IN THE STORM

CHIPPED PAINT

Leaning over the edge of my apartment patio window, I watch the tiny cars pass below me. My eyes close as I listen to the soft hum of movement. The breeze at the 19th floor is soft and gentle, not strong like you would expect. The air is warm, and the scent is sweet, like gardenias in full bloom. The Honolulu city noise fills the air, which is strangely calming. It was an ordinary day in Hawaii, but the moment was not.

My arms stretch across the metal frame enclosing my patio and I'm frozen in the moment. I'm still, numb, and almost paralyzed throughout my body. My mind was lost and tired from all the thoughts. My eyes open towards the vibrant orange skyline overlooking the beach and I take a deep breath. As tears rolled down my cheeks, I knew, this would be my future.

Sitting down into my wicker chair, I reflected on the past two years. Moving from the Big Island of Hawaii to Oahu was a huge choice but the right move for my career. I knew if I wanted to be successful as a makeup artist, I had to move to the main island of Oahu and move up the ranks to the trainer position. Still, that initial year separated from my partner took a toll on our relationship. It chipped away at us like crappy paint on walls. Peel by peel, argument by argument we were piling up flakes of paint, not knowing how much we stripped away. Living separately was unexpected and we did what we could, but it was hard. When we finally moved back in with each other, we thought things were okay. They weren't. But I continued on like everything was.

Now, here I was. At this point of emotional despair on my patio. Anxiety ridden and feeling like I was just repainted over. I look down at my large belly and feel a swift kick, almost like she knew I needed a friend. I rub my tummy and cry. Then laugh. Then cry and laugh while wiping away tears. Why the hell am I laughing? Humor has always helped me cope, even when it seemed inappropriate.

I really believed I did things the right way. Dated for a few years, graduated college, got married, and *then* planned a family. In my mind, that was what you were supposed to do. That would ensure a happy, successful future. Life, however, does not care what you have planned. It does not reward you for the path you took or value how long it took you to get there. It does not weigh one choice over the other as "the right way" and sure as hell does not ensure one path is less painful than another. My body felt like lead as I agonized through this. My mind, usually fluttered with thoughts, began to surrender.

I was finally embracing the unknown. Not because I wanted to, but because I knew I had to, for me and my baby. I was allowing myself to see a different way of life rather than the one I carefully crafted. Holding on made me cling to a past, but letting go made me face a future. A new future, one that I had no idea how to navigate. I accepted I was no longer in control, and it was terrifying. Wiping away tears, I took another deep breath and told myself: things end, shit happens, and you know what? Life moves on, and so must I.

SORRY NOT SORRY

As a college student, I was a lot of fun to be around. I was the only female club DJ on the island and would occasionally rock the mic as a radio personality. I hated the sound of my voice on air but tried to embrace the deeper tone people complimented me on. On most evenings you could find me with a 40-ounce beer in one hand and something to smoke in the other. We'd stay up late bar hopping till the early mornings, often choosing Jack 'n Box since there were few places open at 4 a.m. I really didn't care what I ate, though I was very aware of how I looked. I hid behind my humor, loud hair, and bubbly personality, but inside, I felt my shame.

I graduated with a bachelor's in health and physical education but lived a life of overindulgences and unhealthy behavior. My degree awarded me the title of somewhat knowledgeable in the realm of health, but in actuality, I practiced none of the little I knew. Knowing what to do and actually doing it, would you believe, makes a difference.

I had not really committed to working out since tearing a ligament in my knee at age 20. After that traumatic experience, I stayed away from almost every physical activity I did. Up until that point I was an avid Tahitian dancer and basketball athlete. But everything came to a halt the minute I heard that tendon snap like a tree branch in a game. I was afraid of my injury. I was afraid of the extreme pain I felt. And because of that, I never had courage to return back to the physical activities I loved.

Year after year, I packed on more weight. It happened slowly but steadily. One day, I was scanning through pictures I printed on my recent trip to the Mexican pyramids and stopped at one. My smile soon turned somber as I looked at the photo longer. My shorts were high, high enough to go over my waist to hide what I hated. The length was long, long enough to cover any dimples I loathed on my thighs. The shirt was large, large enough to not grab onto my high waist shorts which would accentuate my wide midsection. As I stared at that photo, I saw a vibrant young woman who was trying so hard to hide herself. How did I get to this point?

At 27, I prepared to have my first child. I knew if I started to conceive while being this unhealthy, I would struggle after pregnancy. So, I quit everything. I quit anything that would harm my body and thus harm my future baby. I wasn't perfect, but just the smallest step of actually thinking before I ate made a huge difference. My health was moving in the right direction and the weight started coming back down. *Not long after finding out I was pregnant, my family received shocking news. My father was diagnosed with stage 3 colon cancer.*

My father was the last person I ever thought would be diagnosed with cancer. He was not overweight, sick, or had any underlying health issues. He took care of his body, even waking up at 4 a.m. to go to the gym before heading to work. He bought books on tai chi and kettlebell strength training, and he knew the importance of exercise. His cancer diagnosis shocked us all.

I, like many daughters, was a daddy's girl. Not only were we close, but we were so alike. Especially when it came to what we liked to eat. We ordered the same meals and always enjoyed the same kind of snacks. So, when my father's oncologist told him that nutrition played a big part in cancer, I was terrified.

I was in my third trimester, dealing with the thought of my father dying, while going through a separation. I developed anxiety, often having panic attacks at the worst times. Once where a carefree young lady stood, now stood a fearful, broken woman. My future felt out of my control. I found help from a marriage family therapist (MFT), and with time, she helped me accept what I already knew. That I cannot control what will happen. I cannot live to find answers to questions I might never have the answers for. What was important was the present. What I could control is what *I* could do. I now had a family history of cancer and imagining my child growing up without her mother shook something in me. My mental and physical self needed to heal. It needed to venture the unknown with courage, compassion, and conviction. It wasn't easy and almost every step of the way felt foreign. But I took it head on with the support of my friends and family around me.

I made sure I went out and did things even though I didn't always feel like it. I went to events with friends and hobbled my rotund figure all the way up the Ward Theatre stairs to watch movies. My friends and I enjoyed many nights eating out in Waikiki discussing how the baby might look, sound, or act. Focusing on her made it easier for me to push forward because I had more to think about than just me. After my realization on the patio where I surrendered to my future, life seemed to be moving forward. Not without pain or agony, but forward. Some days seemed like I made traction towards healing, and some just felt like a haze. The kind of haze that seems like there is no end in sight and you'll just drift on forever. The death of a marriage is devastating. One that was compounded by the future of being a single parent. Something I was not prepared for. In the midst of all of this, I would often sit on my open patio and talk to my belly. I would tell her how wonderful things will be when she gets here, and how so many people will be happy to hold her. I knew she could hear me, and that bond was strong. My daughter was my savior and my strength. She kept me grounded and hopeful for the future. I picked myself up for her and pushed through because I wasn't going to be sorry anymore.

DON'T GET MAD, GET BETTER

I wish I could say I embraced the new mommy body, but who am I kidding. I was a month postpartum, single, and trying to accept all of who I was now. Fresh stretch marks, baby weight, and years of inactivity lead towards feeling really insecure about my body. My identity had been shattered, broken, and scattered everywhere, and now I was unsure of what pieces went where. Not only that but I was still very aware how awful my nutrition was for the last ten years. If there was one thing my father's cancer allowed me to realize is how short and meaningful life can be. I needed to take better care of my health and I needed to be a better example to my daughter.

Once I slapped on my big girl panties, I was determined. Something in me clicked in a way it never had. I was angry. I was angry that I let myself get to this point. This point of feeling so low and utterly vulnerable. My parents raised me to be a strong independent woman, and where was that woman now? Sure, I was independent, I didn't need any financial help, but I sure was not feeling like the strong woman I knew I was. Fire grew in me every day as I became aware of my potential again and I embraced all the challenges to get there. My life had been turned upside down in less than a year, but now I felt a sense of clarity as I embraced this health and fitness journey.

Day by day, I moved towards my goal. Some days I was strong and motivated, other days I collapsed from being so overwhelmed. I had one vision, get in shape. I wasn't sure what that would look like, but I was learning something new about health and fitness every day. I started buying fitness magazines at the grocery store and researching all the latest nutrition information. I'd cut out images of the fitness models I admired and tape them to my fridge, and every time I passed my fridge, I was reminded to make a better choice. The South Beach diet was still big back then, so I grabbed the first book I saw and gave it a try. Within a few weeks, I lost 10 pounds. My clothes fit better, and I was feeling more vibrant and energized. I could see the fruits of my labor and it was rewarding. Once I got down to the weight I thought I wanted, I realized I still wasn't that happy with my body.

Years of playing sports made me think I had more muscle than I had. Once I stripped away the layers of fluff, I realized I don't have much there! I admired the shape and silhouette of the fitness models' bodies on my fridge and knew I needed to do what they did, lift weights. But working out while being a single mother of an infant was hard. I worked in sales which meant irregular work shifts. I was also part-time which meant half the pay I used to make, and not to mention trusting someone (other than my family friend who watched her during work) with my newborn. So what did I do? I dusted off the single 20-pound dumbbell I had in the corner of my apartment and started training at home.

My mother always said, "necessity is the mother of invention," and I took that to heart.

I did everything you could possibly do with that dumbbell. I sat and pressed it over my head, I held it and squatted with it, I held it with both hands and rowed it, and I eventually even one-arm bench-pressed it. I figured out everything I could to create some sort of "workout" feel with my dumbbell. In the beginning, it was hard because it was too heavy for me to do anything with one arm, but I tried using two hands and incorporating different ways of doing a certain exercise. The times I worked out were also all over the place. Some days were normal and I could open up the patio windows for a cool breeze through the apartment, while other days I trained at midnight because of the holiday season. I didn't care, I made it happen. Sometimes I would pick up my daughter late at night, tuck her into bed, close my "private" room divider and workout right there two feet from her. I was so determined to become a better me, nothing could make me waver.

Eventually I was gifted the best piece of equipment I ever had, the Body by Jake Tower 200. What is the Body by Jake Tower 200 you say? Well, only the finest piece of banded equipment you can snap on a door! Easy to install with no footpace, its three tension band system hung from the top of my front door. With not much space in a less than 500-foot apartment, this was golden. The Tower 200 came with a large poster of exercises you could do in 11 minutes a day to get shredded like its endorser, Randy Couture. Its tag line was "11 minutes, no excuses. Get bigger, harder, stronger." I can't say I got much harder or bigger, but I sure got stronger. This thing was amazing! I learned so much about creating tension to maximize what I had because I was limited on what I could do. Three different band tensions means I could vary the intensity, but sometimes the next jump was just too damn hard. Imagine trying to push a pair of bands in front of you, only to get stuck abruptly mid rep as if Randy Couture was pulling me back yelling, "Hey! You ain't that strong yet!" So, like my 20-pound dumbbell, I improvised. I held reps longer or made them really slow in order to make it harder. I squeezed harder at the top of the motion or let it go slowly. I did exercises back-to-back and tried to keep the intensity up. I did the best I could with what I had and you know what? It was good enough. It was good enough to help me start changing the shape of my body and it was good enough to help me become more confident about it too. People could see the change in me and it surprised me. People I hadn't seen in months asked me what I was doing, what I was eating, what happened. They complimented me, and it felt good. As I continued on my journey, people would reach out to me for advice and ask me tips on eating. After some time, I found love for helping people who might be going through similar struggles as I did, and it brought new life to my health and fitness journey.

MYSPACE

It's 2009. Facebook just came out, but really wasn't huge yet. Myspace was dominating the social webs and I, like many people in the early 2000s, had an account. Myspace was unique in that you could change your backgrounds or add music to your account so that your page could really speak to your personality. You could also add your "likes" and "dislikes." There were little customizable aspects that I think they did well on, things we really can't do with Facebook. Don't get me wrong, I'm under no impression Myspace was better than Facebook or else it would still be here, but, there were things about it that I'm probably nostalgic for.

Following my separation, I did what any newly divorced angry woman does, changed her status to SINGLE. In no time at all direct messages came rolling in. Each with their own cheesy pickup lines. Things like "Hey baby, saw your profile and you looking fine. Wanna chat?" Or "Hey cutie wassup you single?" Really? Am I single? You know I'm single, that's how you found me. Little did I know that people hook up through Myspace. I had been so out of the dating loop, I never realized people actually search for single people in the area, like the precursor to the dating apps we see today. One by one I would open and delete. Last thing I was trying to do was meet a guy on Myspace.

Then one day I opened an interesting message. The sender said hi very politely and talked about just moving to Hawaii. I scanned through it as I did the others, with as much cynicism as Joan Crawford, trying hard not to roll my eyes the minute I opened the message. But then, within a few lines, I stopped. I was a little perplexed and went back over what I just read. The sender went on to insult my favorite movies. Remember that part of Myspace where you can customize your likes? Well, this jerk read that I liked all the X-Men movies, even the last one. Then he proceeded to tell me the first ones were good, but the last X-Men was awful and how could I like it. Totally taken back, I thought, who does that? Insults someone as a way to hit on them? I noticed his profile picture was of him and a baby. The curiosity got the best of me and I clicked on his page.

It opened up to a very cool Transformers background. I've always been into sci-fi and could enjoy a good Transformers theme. In his profile photo, he was smiling holding his daughter on his shoulder. She was so small and cute and he looked so happy holding her up, the photo was precious. I kept scrolling and paused at his "Likes" section. Each "like" had an accompanying photo that said the following:

I like to "Party" (insert dumb photo), "Puke" (insert gross photo), and "Pee" (insert dumb and gross photo).

Hell. To. The. No. What? This man is trippen! What woman in her right mind would look at the profile section and think, "hmm he looks like fun!" What a letdown, cause he was actually cute. I muddled around his page a bit more and then went on to write him back. I wasn't interested in him but couldn't hurt jabbing back at him. I told him he was wrong and that he must have poor taste in movies, but I won't hold it against him. I complimented his Transformers background and said he had a cute daughter. It looked like our girls were about the same age. I ended with some niceties and that was that.

After a few months, I decided to put myself out there. I dated a bit, but nothing major. I had some friends that told me about eHarmony and I thought, why not. As a new mom, I was home a lot. Believe or not, you won't find a lot of eligible bachelors sitting on your couch with baby puke on their shirt. I also wanted to be straight up with any guy I dated for real. I wanted to be with someone who would accept me and my daughter. I wasn't going to waver. And, I had a checklist of who I was not interested in:

1. No kids. I know it's hypocritical, but I thought, I'm already adding in our dynamic, why add more kids?
2. No military. I just wasn't into the "they look so good in uniform" thing and my few interactions with military men were usually at a bar, and usually not appealing.
3. Not younger than me. I needed someone mature.
4. No Latinos. Also hypocritical since I am Latina. But my experience with the good looks is that they can also come from a flirtatious personality. Been there, done that.

I know that this list is riddled with stereotypes and assumptions, but at the time I thought I was safeguarding my future. I thought staying away from this list would help me find the right guy or at least make things easy to rule out the ones who might not be right. Time went on and eHarmony didn't really pan out. I liked how it worked, and I almost took the next step with someone, but last minute I decided not to. Would you believe, through all this time, the Transformers guy would message me. He was always friendly and easy to chat online with. We came from very different backgrounds but had a lot of the same interests. Both a little nerdy, both parents of infants and both recently separated. I found solace in our chats; it was nice to talk about new parent things with someone who was going through the same struggles and joys I was. He was up late with the baby as I was sometimes, and it was nice to chat with someone at times when it feels very lonely. Not lonely physically, because your child is there with you, but lonely with companionship. I could see how people stay with someone even though it might feel like roommates.

We grew to know each other over the following months and though we never physically met, I liked him. I made a friend and I learned that's hard to do as you become an adult. One day he told me he was going to the mall I worked at to take pictures with his daughter. We decided to meet at the little coffee kiosk upstairs from my work before I started my shift. I walked around the area a bit, hoping to run into him coming in from one of the entrances. Waiting, I glanced through the windows of the neighboring jewelry shops and admired the newest sparkly additions to the store. I could never afford anything in this place but always imagined what it would look like to own something there. Then, a reflection from behind me caught my eye. It was him. As I turned around, I saw him pushing a pink stroller ahead of himself while quickly pulling his pants up. I'm not sure why that memory stayed with me, but I guess I thought it was cute. He was cute. It was a sweet dad moment. I waved and smiled at him as I made my way across the walkway to the other side of the mall. He quickly caught eyes with me, smiled, and waved back. I was anxious, I didn't really expect to be.

But he was cuter than I thought he would be. I had seen pictures of him, but you never know when you actually meet someone. We made our way to the second floor and picked a table to sit at. I went to order my coffee and asked him what he would like. He said "Oh, no thank you. I don't drink coffee." What? Why would you want to meet at a coffee spot if you don't even drink coffee? Because I suggested it and he was being polite. So here I was, my coffee in hand and him with his daughter. She was so precious. She had the cutest pink dress on with a bow headband around her little bald head. She was a few months older than my daughter but about the same size. He was so natural with her, it was nice. He wasn't as chatty in person as he was online, and I felt like I was talking too much trying to fill the silence. We hung out for about 15 minutes and then I headed to work. He went on to take pictures with his daughter and I started my shift.

Right before I walked on the floor, he texted me "you looked beautiful today". I felt all warm and fuzzy inside, kinda like riding over a little hill.

I told him "Thanks. You looked cute too. It was nice to finally meet you in person".

That 15-minute coffee led to dinner and movies, which led to seeing each other almost every day. He would sometimes drive an hour to chat with me for my 15-minute break, then stay in town till I finished work so we could hang out. He was a persistent man. There were many times I told him "okay well if I see you then I see you," not thinking he was that serious. But he was, and he showed it all the time. He was fun and easy to be with. We got along so well. Our time together wasn't filled partying at the club like others our age, but rather video games and home movies. We'd hang out all the time at one of our places since we had the kids. Day by day my heart opened up to this man without knowing it. I was once so bitter and angry, and he made me soft again. I laughed all the time and he allowed me to feel loved again. I was scared, he was scared. But we trusted each other and never looked back.

Today, the man who I met on Myspace, who had a child, who was in the Army, who is younger than me and who is Latino, is my husband of almost 11 years. Deven and I have an amazing marriage and an even deeper friendship. He's a devoted husband and loves me beyond words. We've traveled the U.S. together with our two little girls in hand and even had another little girl together. My heart grew exponentially becoming Danika's mother, and I would have made the worst mistake of my life if I decided not give him a chance because of some dumb list. See, in a time when my life felt so out of control, I was trying to control it again with this list. This list was my standards and I wasn't going to lower my standards. But they really weren't standards, they were fears. Pain points I hoped I wouldn't relive or have to live. As I grew to love Deven, I could see how wrong I was, about a lot. He was impulsive and I was calculated. He decides with his gut, and I questioned mine. I thought about things for a while before making a decision while he would say the first answer that came to him. I admired his assurance towards decisions because in the end, he wasn't afraid of what would happen, even if it didn't work out. I learned to not fear taking more chances in life again. I still was scared when we moved from state to state or when he deployed to Iraq for a year, not knowing how it would end up. But I felt secure that I would be okay. That the worse had happened already, and I weathered that storm. That I had the strength to not let fear hold me back from anything again, especially love. They say people are more open to change following an emotional or pivotal event in their life and all I had been through really put things into perspective. I was enjoying our life right now, in the present, and not worrying about the future. I followed my heart, and as cheesy as that sounds, it has got me far.

BEYOND THE 6-PACK

I want you to imagine for a minute this is you. You are nervously standing in front of a mirror with nothing but a skimpy rhinestone studded bathing suit, big hoop earrings, and 4-inch clear heels. And no, you're not a stripper. Your long, flowy, oversprayed hair is a combination of Farrah Fawcett and Kim Kardashian's, and your makeup looks so good RuPaul would be jealous.

This was the day you've been waiting for.

You turn around and check out your toned, shredded body, striking your best Instagram pose, but all you feel is exhausted and hungry. For the last four weeks you've eaten less than 1,000 calories and have done two hours of cardio on top of your strength training workouts just to have the lowest body fat possible. You haven't had your period in two months, but that's okay because that means your body fat is really low. You've been dieting and training hard for five months for this one day to step on stage in the best shape of your life and all you can think is... I'm too fat.

You tell yourself "Hike up the suit! You need to hide the love handles so the judges don't see" and "Don't tie the suit too hard, it will squeeze the back fat." You suck it in, you suck it in and turn, then you suck it in, turn, and stop breathing. Perfect. You tell yourself you shouldn't have eaten the extra cucumber and salad dressing every day. You should have done a harder cardio session these last couple weeks and did an extra cardio session on Thanksgiving because that fat is just hanging around your tummy. You shamefully look around and all you can see is other women like yourself, except they look better.

You tell yourself they were more disciplined, they probably didn't cheat as often as you did, and they didn't have the family curse of love handles. You feel defeated before you've even walked onto the stage.

This story, my story, is not a unique story among women in fitness. Besides the glittery suit and spray tan, this story is not far from the narrative many women tell themselves in the mirror. That our bodies, no matter where they're at, no matter the journey they came to get there, is just not good enough. I thought I had come so far over the years, but I really hadn't. Sure, I was proud of my body I worked for, but I realized at almost every great milestone in my fitness journey I also was highly critical and disappointed with some part of my physique. Lost the baby weight? Damn, why's my butt so flat? Fit into a size 4? Yikes why are my legs so skinny! Finished my first fitness competition! UGH, I was the fattest of all the women on stage. I soon learned that this is what Dr. Lindsay Kite of the nonprofit organization "Beauty

Redefined" calls self-objectification.

Self-objectification is the monitoring of your body from an outsider's perspective, aka, self-consciousness. It's the voice in your head that talks negatively about your body and is fixated on appearance. Much of the time, without even knowing it. It's conversations like "Ugh, those shorts show all my cottage cheese" or "I need more concealer, everyone's going to think I'm so tired with these bags." So why is this so bad? I'm sure some of you might be thinking, well, it's true!

Approximately 91% of women are unhappy with their bodies and resort to dieting to achieve their ideal body shape. Dr. Kite says studies show girls who engage with self-objectification perform worse in reading and comprehension, can't run as fast, and CAN'T LIFT heavy weights. That those who thought about themselves more in terms of their appearance were more likely to be ashamed of their bodies. And secretly, I was ashamed.

Competing in bodybuilding was a goal of mine ever since the first day I cut out my fitness models picture to hang on my fridge. Every year, I took a step closer to that dream as I increased my strength training knowledge and eventually became a personal trainer. I would admire the physiques so much and knew that they were the epitome of "health and fitness." Admittedly, I liked that I could try something others found hard. I took on this challenge and it felt good knowing I was not "average." I'd meal prep each week with my tilapia and asparagus, apple and cheese stick, whey shakes with creatine, and cycle my carbs throughout the months. If you broke it down, I was dieting for more than half the year to slowly get my body fat down to the right percentage to be on stage.

Eventually, I came to a realization. That for me, competing in bodybuilding only heightened my fixation. It allowed me to mask the insecure obsession as "dedication" and "discipline." I thought it was a healthy, noble goal to physically push my body and mind. And in some aspects, it was. I learned a lot about routine, diet manipulation, and stage presence. I loved being on the stage and loved the art of posing. But I was judging how fit I was on how I looked rather than my actual health. My actual health was awful. Missing your period at my age is your body's way of telling you you're not healthy enough to house a baby. I couldn't look at food without seeing a number, and I thought about how my body looked almost all day. I was working out with the intention to "fix" something that I hated about myself and that came with a whole host of baggage, like negative self-talk, hyper-monitoring of my body, and comparison, either with other people or with my imaginary future self. I struggled with wanting to look fit and healthy, and actually BEING healthy. But after that last competition in New York, I realized I couldn't do it anymore. I was burnt out and needed to find why I loved fitness in the first place.

Let me tell you what I did:

- I made clear intentions about my fitness. I had to have fun training again instead of loathing it.
- I stopped counting calories and macronutrients and started to introduce some freedom in my eating without judgment.
- I stopped following bodybuilding/fitspo-ish people on my social media. Every once in a while, I would sit and stare and compare and it would just pull me back mentally at a time when I wasn't as resilient as I am now.
- I stopped competing in bodybuilding and started training with the intention of what my body could do rather than how I could make it look better. And for me, that was going back to powerlifting. It's a sport of lifting weights that, for the most part, is objective. You lift the weight or you don't. *No one is telling me my glutes need to be tighter.*
- I actively resisted self-objectification. As hard as it was, I tried to not let myself speak badly about my appearance.
- I started training with a small group of women and found myself laughing and sweating and having the greatest time challenging myself physically. It was amazing.

If we shift our focus from solely to what we look like to more about what our bodies can do, I find we could truly achieve a better level of health and fitness. The irony here is that NOT trying to change how I looked actually changed how I looked. I found myself enjoying how my body changed and feeling confident with being the trainer who didn't necessarily have veins on her stomach anymore, but could squat, bench, and deadlift a lot of weight. I let go of the judgment I had built the last couple of years and started to feel comfortable just being me.

Now, many years later, I own a successful strength gym with my husband called Core Strength & Performance, have been a competitive powerlifter for almost 10 years, have a fantastic team of online and in-person powerlifters I coach (mostly women by the way), host one of the only podcasts about women in powerlifting called *The Future Is Female Powerlifting*, and get to be featured on great pages such as *Girls Who Powerlift* speaking about my life journey.

This process is a continuous ongoing step towards body image resilience. Some days I'm bulletproof, some days I'm really hard on myself. But the difference is now when I look in the mirror, I don't see mostly flaws, I see strength. I see a mom who can roller-skate with her kids to the park without hesitation and then whip up a batch of cookies so we can all share together, I see a wife who is less insecure and feels sexy most of the time rather than critical. And when I look around my competitions now, I don't compare, I'm inspired. I'm surrounded by men and women of all ages, all sexes and races who are all just trying to be the strongest version of themselves. Not one person is thinking about my belly squeezing out of my lifting belt, only how much I lift.

WHAT MATTERS

As I write this, I'm staring at a picture of my grandfather that sits on top of my computer desk. The frame is black, the background is white and framed inside are two things. On the left is a small 2.5 x 3 black-and-white photo of my grandfather in his 20s. He's in an Army uniform, has a mic in his hands, and headphones on. He's casually leaned over with his arm resting on top of what looks like the inside of a vehicle, and his legs crossed just slightly over each other comfortably. The picture always reminded me how cool he was without even trying. Not like us nowadays, carefully crafting the image we want others to see. Making sure we have the right lighting or a good angle. He stood there for the photo and probably just looked up. Next to this picture is a blue Post-it note. One of the only things I have left that has his writing on it. The note reads "This is for Heidi. Paid on death. 8/2002, 10 years." This was the note that was attached to a monetary deposit left to me by my grandfather. He died January 4th, 2000.

Almost 20 years later, I have kept this note as a reminder. A reminder of what's really important in my life. The money, it's gone. Probably spent on bills, those acquired by a second-year college student. I'm sure it made good use at the time, but really, it didn't matter. Taking a step back and looking at my life throughout the years, it's only been a sliver of something inconsequential. I'd give any amount of money to be able to spend five more minutes with my grandpa. That time I had with him, that is what matters. Those moments where I'm present with my kids laughing and making cookies, that matters. Time shared with my friends laughing about who's getting older, that's what matters. The way I love and care for myself as I age, that matters. I look at my grandfather's photo and love his big cheeks and wrinkled face. And it reminds me to love mine just as much, though I'm constantly shown images to nip and tuck what's sagging. This photo is a reminder, though I strive for success and achievement, never to be blinded by wanting more. It's easy to get caught up in having more or just being more. Competing more or expanding the business more because that's what we're often conditioned to do, achieve more because more is better. Getting more has to take energy away from other things. I won't sacrifice attending parties because I'm on a diet or stay inside on a day I told my kids we'd go out because I'm too beat up from training. There are things in life that are nonnegotiable for me now, and I won't put work or competing over what matters most anymore. It took some time learning, but after trying, failing, and getting back up, the answer becomes very clear.

REFLECTIONS

REFLECTIONS

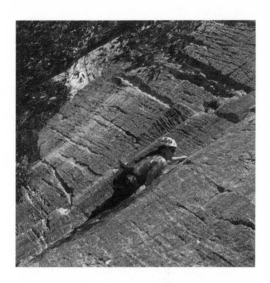

ANNIE GIBBINS
AUSTRALIA

Annie Gibbins, transformation queen, internationally recognized corporate CEO, keynote speaker, podcast host, and creator of the MAGIC Transformation program and mastermind series, philanthropist, wife, and mother of five. A lot of titles for one woman, but not surprising when you consider a woman who has high levels of curiosity and a passion to raise other women so they can be more, achieve more, and earn more just by being themselves. With academic and professional accolades over the past 30 years including growing and transforming health and education businesses across Australasia, Annie also has a Master of Education, a Bachelor of Nursing, Lean Six Sigma, Cert. IV Fitness, and a MAICD.

Annie Gibbins is one of the top women in the corporate world when it comes to female leadership. With her tried and tested MAGIC Transformation program, a clearly defined methodology and framework, she calls out limiting beliefs, clarifies her clients' purpose, and develops strong business practices, quickly turning dreams and goals into mind-blowing reality.

Her fascinating life story is shared in a biography about her and her rise to the top in *Becoming Annie: A Biography of a Curious Woman*. Her podcast, *Memoirs of Successful Women*, is a window into the passion she has for celebrating other women and guiding them into living a life with purpose, passion, and authenticity.

To discover more about Annie, please visit https://anniegibbins.com

CHAPTER FIVE

CREATE YOUR OWN STAGE

Reading the opening chapter of my biography, I got swept up and transported back to the very moment my dreams were shattered. When I was a young girl, I had imagined my name in lights, on billboards around the world, and standing center stage captivating every audience I had the honor and the privilege to perform for.

I am pretty sure there have been times when you have imagined yourself so excited and full of life that you can't wait for the next opportunity to reveal itself and invite you in. You have had, or currently have, big dreams, a big smile, a cheesy grin, and a knowing smirk etched permanently on your face. When you let your mind linger, it radiates pure joy which resonates through every fiber of your being. You will probably have this knowing deep inside, that you are destined for greatness. I know I did! Add to the smile that frown of determination, resilience, and focus, and it doesn't matter how long you have had this dream, this goal, or this vision of you stepping up onto the winners podium; it's an excitement which is impossible to contain and needs to burst forth.

The smile on your face has given your facial muscles the best workout possible, so much so your face aches in the best possible way. You bow to your audience, who are raising the roof with their thunderous applause, your heart overflowing with joy, not quite believing this is all possible, but going with it anyway.

If you are anything like me, you know you are here to change the world, and this belief in yourself lights you up in each and every moment, and it shows. You are radiant, your eyes sparkling, and you are so enthusiastic you've almost reached the point of excitement where only dogs can hear your voice. People love being around you because you are so positive, and sometimes you just don't get why everyone is not this happy. For you to be reading this book, you know the immense value of being able to read stories that inspire and empower you in your unique and special life journey.

There are those moments when all your dreams have possibly been shattered, and the people you love most in the world are the ones responsible. The ones you were led to believe would be the ones cheering you on the loudest. The ones you thought were helping you to achieve every dream you ever had, even the fantasy dreams of a young girl who would wake up to discover her wings were all sparkly and full of glitter and rainbows. It happened to me too, as you can probably tell by that last sentence.

I had a pretty normal family life, and I am the youngest of three children, the only girl, and like most sisters, I was on the receiving end of daily taunts from my brothers. My dad had his own pharmacy business, and I idolized him. I was a proper daddy's girl. My relationship with my mom was the exact opposite to what I had with my dad.

With dreams of being a world-famous ballerina, I trained like my life depended on it. Every day was ballet day, but Friday nights, oh they were just the highlight of my week! I could hardly contain myself and would get very excited and gather up my things, put my beautiful tutu and soft ballet cardigan in my ballet bag ready to impress the world, or rather just my ballet teacher. I would have my hair tightly up in a bun, and my baby pink tights underneath the soft pink body. It was time to shine like the radiant star on a global stage that I believed I would one day become, and secretly believed I already was.

I was eight years old and ready to take on the world of ballet. With youthful confidence, I felt ready to take to the stage at any given moment, joy bursting from every part of me, ready to shine my gorgeous smile out to the back row of any theater of any size!

The world would see me dance, applaud me in gratitude for my awe-inspiring talent and for telling the most beautiful, romantic love stories in the most graceful and silent of ways. I was going to be a famous ballerina just like my Russian-born Aunt Anna Volkova, who danced on stages from Paris to Havana with the Ballet Russes. I dreamed it, I believed it, and I was going to do it and live it!

That was until the moment I excitedly told my grandma, "I'm going to be a famous ballerina just like Auntie Ania." And with a chuckle and a wry smile on her face, my grandmother delivered words which shattered my childhood dream into a thousand tiny pieces. No words of encouragement or dream building, just a soul-destroying moment that made the anger rise up within me. I remember the tears falling down my face and going to my mother. She would surely be as equally shocked and upset at my grandma's response.

"You'll never believe what Mama said to me! She even made me cry! She said that I will never be a world-famous ballerina like Aunt Ania. She told me I have legs like an elephant!"

But what I heard next would be equally devastating and would lay the foundations of years of self-doubt.

"Darling, Mama is right. You will not be a world-famous ballerina. You don't have legs like an elephant... but you do have a lot of puppy fat. You don't have the body to be a ballerina." Delivered in a soothing way, graced by the word "Darling" at the beginning of the sentence, as if that would make it less painful to hear, my mother sealed the fate on my glorious life of dance.

I was in shock, had never felt so deflated and devastated! I didn't know it was possible to feel this sad. I had always had a shiny excitedness about me, and now I felt as though someone had reached into my body and pulled the plug on the energy that lit me up every day. I was distraught. How could they say these things to me?

I was left feeling fat and ugly, not daring to dream for the fear of it being crushed right there in front of me again. The very person who should have been there to turn fears and doubts into courage and confidence had been the one to dim my light and fill me with dread.

Deciding never to go to ballet ever again, having formed the opinion that I was a terrible dancer, and definitely too fat to belong in a room of dancers, I went home and announced that I was taking up swimming instead.

With swimming, my body would be hidden underneath the water, so no one would see my fat legs, fat body, and the clumsiness of an elephant.

Taking to the water and training every Saturday with a midweek session thrown in for good measure, I felt free. I could wobble and jiggle as much as I liked, no one could see my body once I was in the water, but I still felt the wobbles, and the jiggles, and I still believed I was fat. While I had the power to become a competitive swimmer, my negative self-talk did not allow me to capitalize on any potential, so I used the time swimming to get my asthma under control, to a point, and develop strong arms and shoulders, something which would hold me in good stead in the coming years.

Arriving at high school with my large breasts and curvaceous body enveloped by an unflattering uniform which resembled a sack, my best friend from primary turned away from me to join "The Models"—a group I would never belong to because I was too fat. I was an elephant. I had fat legs. I was fat; puppy fat or not, it still had the word fat at the end of the phrase, and for a young prepubescent girl like myself, using the word fat anywhere in a sentence is never going to be a good idea.

There were many things I wanted to do, like the school drama, but my mother dearest wouldn't allow it as it "would upset my asthma and distract me from my studies." But I didn't realize in these heart-breaking moments that I was alchemizing the strength and determination, the foundation of resilience which would turn me into the hugely successful woman I am today.

It is uncomfortable for me to say that I am hugely successful, because even though I know I am, I am simply Annie. Someone who loves to serve others, someone who loves celebrating others and raising money and awareness for incredible charities such as Glaucoma Australia, of which I am CEO and have been for many years now. I have been chosen to be a keynote speaker at world congresses and summits for a variety of medical, health, and education organizations, and in 2020, I was selected to be one of the board directors for a women's health charity called MRKH.

The knock backs, bullying, and deep sadness I experienced as a child paved the way for me in different ways. I remember returning to my ballet class the week after those awfully hurtful words spoken by my mother and grandmother to watch the girls, to see how they twirled with what seemed like effortless ease. I compared myself and my own journey to theirs; throughout my teens, I continued with the comparison.

This comparison that I felt, combined with a few traumatic events in my family life, led me to develop anorexia nervosa. I would go without food, and the less space I took up, the thinner and weaker I got, the more compliments I received. The more compliments I embraced, the more I thought I must be doing something right, because we only get praise for the good things we do, right? Wrong.

We receive praise from others for a variety of reasons, including when they want something from us, when they want to keep us less than them, when we are less of a threat to them, and when what we are doing makes them feel more powerful or inferior to them. It took me a long time to figure all this out, and even sometimes today I have moments of not feeling worthy enough. In the corporate world, it is known as "imposter syndrome," and yet for me it wasn't so much a self-worth issue as many people experience, it was more of a side effect of my never-ending curiosity about life, people, and the planet.

My insatiable curiosity has led me to create some crazy goals in my life and put myself into some very uncomfortable situations when it comes to being the one in the room who knows the least amount of the topic. I love learning from others; absorbing knowledge from books, experts, and nature; and pushing myself further than ever before.

When I pushed my body to the extreme of anorexia nervosa, I learned a lot about myself, especially when a dear friend went into the hospital with the same condition and nearly died. I snapped out of my destructive behavior really quickly, just like I changed direction from dancing to swimming. I didn't know it then, but my skill for adapting quickly and learning new ways of being was already strong.

I was strong, and over the years the more I cycled around the local area, the more I got out hiking and kayaking in nature, the more I learned about taking care of my body, I realized the value of good health, self-love, and honoring the body I was given. This revelation compounded when I became pregnant with my first set of twins. Yes! I had more than one set of twins! It seemed pushing my body to the extreme of anorexia nervosa was the least demanding thing I could do! I was one of the lucky ones, because anorexia nervosa can really damage your chances of having babies, and not only did my first set of twins prove I hadn't damaged my fertility, but the second set of twins arriving just two years after the first set meant I was apparently super fertile! Scary and exciting all at the same time, and who has two sets of twins? I mean who does that? Not many of us, that's for sure!

During and after having our two sets of twins, two years apart, my husband James and I took more notice of our health. We had been reasonably active and healthy, but with four children in 26 months, we needed to consciously focus on maximizing the quality of our sleep, mindset, communication and energy levels. Now was not a time to compare with anyone else, it was time to be our best self, and that was more than enough.

I am not like the other ladies in this book, I am not your classical proper athlete, but then I get that is just another limitation or belief that is lingering in my subconscious mind. (Here I go getting curious again!) What is a proper athlete anyway? What does it mean to be fit and strong, or simply strong?

Pushing two babies out one after the other, you need a lot of stamina, and a strong determination to just keep going even when you want to quit. Growing two more babies inside of you when running around after toddlers, again it takes a level of emotional, physical, and mental strength to get through each day.

Over the years, I became curious about what it takes to be the best version of myself, personally, professionally, and as a wife, mother, sister, and friend. I wanted more out of life. I wanted to lead my children and other women by example, because other than my grandmothers, who have always been my biggest inspiration, there was never anyone I really had as a role model.

Growing up, the only women ever really spoken about as great women were Mother Theresa and, in the 1980s, Margaret Thatcher, the British Prime Minister. We had the likes of Marie Curie, Rosa Parks, and tennis stars like Martina Navratilova, runners like Zola Budd, and ice skaters such as Tonya Harding, but where were the women in business, female business owners? My dream was to become a businesswoman and having been told by my dad that I wasn't strong enough at math to make that a possibility, I was again feeling deflated, but determined. I was so determined that I even wrote on a piece of paper "I have higher-level managerial skills" and stuck it to the fridge freezer door, which even today provides my family and friends with giggles and laughter at given opportunities.

Getting curious about my future career at a time of being a mother to four children all under five, I began to get excited, but also a sense of overwhelm. Could I really do this? I started studying, taking time out before my classes to go and read a magazine or a book in the café close by to my evening classes. It felt so naughty, but really good too. Not long after my university degree finished, James and I found out we are to become parents again. Slightly freaked out by this news, well… more than a bit freaked out to be honest, because would we have twins again? Or would this time we be blessed with one? Or maybe three? We were both excited to get to the first ultrasound scan to find out and also very nervous. In the back of my mind, I started to wonder if I would ever be more than just a mother, and isn't that an interesting phrase "Just a mother," as if it is a lowly job and not a role in society to be celebrated. James was more worried about another set of twins, and God forbid triplets! Thankfully, when we looked at the monitor screen, there was only one baby, and the relief swept over us both, for very different reasons.

Back home, I put my "higher-level managerial skills" to great use with the support of a loving husband who was, and still is a very hands-on dad, which even as little as 20 years ago was almost unheard of. I became super organized and the best project manager there ever was, well as I knew how to be, and I felt that was pretty great!

Sunday afternoon was a very special time for me as I got to go sailing with my beloved father, a man whose health over the years had been slowly ravaged by a brain tumor. It didn't really have anything to do with the sailing, I just enjoyed being on the water. It was being with my dad and being out in nature which gave me clarity in the moments of crazy, gave me the air to breathe and connect with God in prayer. Being a mother to five children, having a very sick father, and creating a successful career while studying and being a great wife meant that finding time for me was, at the beginning, really hard, but over the years I realized it was so important, so much so I wrote a book on it! I have always had an unwavering belief in God and releasing whatever I couldn't figure out, or feel like I couldn't handle, up to Him. It was for me an act of trust, worship, and faith. Trusting everything would work itself out, not stressing about anything, which had a really great bonus because it also helped me defy the aging process! Who knew that learning to be still, being regular in prayer, getting out in nature and appreciating all of God's creations, breathing in the fresh air, exploring the mind, pushing while also respecting the body, and connecting with fellow humans would be better than the most expensive collagen boosters? But for me it worked.

As my children got older and became more and more independent, I was able to have more time for myself, and with James. James is my absolutely gorgeous husband, my best friend, and we get up to all sorts of fun together. Family is really important to both of us, and we are all incredibly close, and while I know many people can say the same, learning to balance everything and give five kids a great life, full of adventure, wasn't easy. We were mid-level managers with the bills everyone else had. We had five kids to buy school uniforms for, to take on holiday, and of course feed. For those of you reading this with kids, you will know how much they eat when they hit puberty, especially the boys! James and I have three boys and two girls, so it was absolutely necessary I harnessed those higher-level managerial skills of mine. Having to budget bills, holidays, and school trips, I became really great at budgeting and making money go as far as it could, skills and knowledge which laid a lot of the foundation skills in my work as a CEO and board director for two health care charities.

Being the mother of two sets of twins two years apart, followed by the blessing of a fifth child, took its toll on my body, and my mental health. My visits to the gym gave me the focus I needed and the results I wanted, but I loved being outdoors. My friend Ilda and I would meet up with our girlfriends for a hike on the weekends, followed by coffee and a chat, and I loved being able to push myself further than I thought possible. As my twin boys got closer to finishing school and the Gibbins tribe became more helpful around the home, I had even more time for myself, so I started looking for my next big challenge. It wasn't enough for me though to just take care of my body, I wanted to be able to give back to the community, help others in the process of helping myself.

I then came across an organization which had been organizing events across Australia since 2009, and with the excitement and a few too many drinks, my colleague Maria and I came up with the idea of completing the 2014 Sydney Coastrek. The Sydney Coastrek is an outdoor trek along the coast, the clue really is in the name with this one, and consisted of varying distances starting from 30 to 60 kilometers. Maria and I set about training for the "big walk" and soon it was time for us girls to tie up our boot laces and get on with it. Little did I know that taking part in the 2014 Sydney Coastrek event would mean that the 30–60-kilometer Team Trekking Challenge was going to be the start of annual fundraising events for me, but I loved it, even though it wasn't an easy hike, and it wasn't just a walk either. Our team had not all trained as per "the plan," so it took us 15 hours to complete, which was plenty of time for a great natter, a good giggle, and a breathtaking walk along 60 kilometers of the most beautiful paths the Sydney region has to offer. I saw my hometown in a completely different way and discovered more about myself and my friends than ever before, and I raised $5000AUD for the Fred Hollows Foundation[1] in the process! The foundation was founded in 1992 by eye surgeon Fred Hollows shortly before he died. He was an incredibly talented surgeon, as well as a social justice activist who was committed to improving eye health for Aboriginals and for those in developing countries such as Eritrea, Nepal, and Vietnam. He was also an instigator of bringing down the cost of eye health care and educating the Indigenous population of all the 19 countries his foundation now operates in, thanks to his widowed wife Gabby carrying out his work after his death. The way in which he and his wife Gabby give back to others is something I really respect and admire about others.

It felt great completing this Coastrek, and I wasn't "just" a mom anymore, and so I registered again and again, and from 2014 to 2019 I have been supported by some really great people, and together we have raised $17,500AUD for the Fred Hollows Foundation. My Bluebirds team has also reduced our time by 5 hours, so we are pretty chuffed by that!

Getting through the 60 kilometers was a great achievement, but being the kind of woman who asks, "Well if I can do that, what else can I do?" I started to look for my next big challenge. My beautiful soul sister Ilda had been planning for months to trek to Ama Dablam Base Camp in Nepal. As I listened to her share about her upcoming adventure, I felt that "excited, full of life, can't wait for the next opportunity to reveal itself and invite you in" moment confront me with full force. While James called it a serious case of FOMO, it made me join her group at the last minute. With the "warm up" along the coast

---

1   https://www.hollows.org/au/home

in Sydney completed, it was time to head 14,993 feet above sea level to the base camp situated 4,570 meters up in the mountains. A whole new level of training and preparation was required, but I did every single requirement on the training plan plus more as I couldn't stand being the weakest link. I also felt fantastic being this fit, and now that I'd gone to all this effort, I promised myself to keep it as I would then be couch ready for any future adventures that came my way.

I loved the way the trek to base camp was designed to take trekkers through the various Sherpa villages. Joining other trekkers, Ilda and I were all set to go and have the adventure of a lifetime. The trek follows the same trail for those on their way to Everest Base Camp, and beyond, and is just so gorgeous with the colors of the sun, snow, and shadows all being blended into one. When we reached Ama Dablam, we could clearly see why it means "mother's necklace" due to the way the hanging glaciers resemble the traditional jewelry worn for centuries by the Sherpa women.

We took lots of photos at various intervals of the breathtaking scenery, and we had a truly amazing time in some of the most rugged landscapes on the planet. My childhood asthma had been the thing to take away my breath at school and in my early twenties, but I never allowed this to stop me then, and I certainly wasn't going to allow it to stop me now! The high altitude and lack of oxygen didn't bother me, probably because I was so taken by the sun shining on the snowy peaks, the incredible blue skies, and the vastness of it all. My hubby James was coincidentally in Nepal at the same time, but he was giving back to the community and helping others on an optical aid trip. When we got back home to Sydney, we started sharing our experiences of Nepal, and before I knew it, James and I were already getting excited about going back the following year to do the Everest Base Camp circuit including the three high passes and beautiful Gokyo Lake together. It was the only way to overcome the hit of loving jealousy he had when seeing all my photos, and it took me all of a millisecond to agree to go back. I was so excited to share this magical experience with my love and knew if I had done it once, I could do it again. Training for it together brought us closer together, and being able to share something we both loved as a couple outside of our children also made us stronger together, as well as physically, mentally, and emotionally strong as individuals.

With a lot of the work I do with Glaucoma Australia, I get to see and hear about some really sad stories, and this can be emotionally draining, as well as truly inspiring. There are people with really positive outcomes, and this can bring tears of joy to my eyes. They have just had their sight saved or repaired and the joy that brings to them and their families makes my heart burst with happiness. Knowing we get to help people keep their sight longer is so rewarding. I get to work with some of the most visionary people (excuse the pun!) and the work they do is incredible. We get to improve the quality of so many people's lives and that is a really great thing to be part of. Sometimes when I feel like I am hitting "The Wall" during one of my coastal treks or out hiking in the mountains, I just remember some of the people who cannot take part in what I am doing, and I feel like I am doing it for them. They get me through it. My children get me through it, knowing that I am leading them by the example of not quitting when things get tough.

One of my favorite memories of trekking is when my soul sister and best friend Ilda and I went on another adventure together: a three-day camping trip to Mount Kosciuszko, Australia's highest mountain. It was in 2018, and we were at 2,228 meters above sea level, and while we were there, we were met with a blizzard, one that reduced visibility to just a few meters. The irony of this situation was not lost on me, and again I felt incredibly blessed to be able to work for an eye care charity and help save other people's sight.

Due to all the training, preparation, and climbing I have done over the years, I am a pretty experienced climber and trekker, so leading Ilda and a few others, I was very confident that we would all be okay. Besides the obvious safety requirements, it was mainly about keeping spirits high, making sure everyone was filled with positivity by encouraging and motivating them (Those higher-level managerial skills of mine come in hand in pretty much every situation!). Once we had made it through the blizzard, we celebrated by trekking a couple of kilometers to the Eagles Nest Pub for a much-needed hot chocolate, and a cheeky Peach Schnapps or two, my favorite sweet spirit. We were all keen to eat a proper meal, because although I am a lover of the great outdoors, I am certainly not a fan of camp food!

One of the things I love to do is celebrate achievements, big or small; it helps keep me, and others, motivated, and if there has been a particularly challenging personal or professional success, then celebrating what we have achieved lifts the mood and helps us see the distance we have all traveled in terms of courage, determination, perseverance, and of course physically.

So as I wrap up this chapter, I encourage you to pursue your dreams, to believe in yourself, and to ignore the cruel words of another, because I may not have made it to the world stage in my ballet tutu dancing to the greats such as Swan Lake, but I do get to appear on a variety of different stages around the world speaking about the things which really truly matter. I help women be more, achieve more, and earn more by activating the strength, determination and power that lies within them, waiting to be unleashed so their true essence can reveal itself. There are no limits on what is truly possible. We all have the strength necessary to keep going when things get tough and achieve abundance in this life. We just need to believe it is possible, and I mean truly believe where you see yourself standing on that podium, hearing the thunderous applause, and grinning from ear to ear.

Whatever challenge you are facing, just know that whatever life throws at you, whether that is glaucoma or another health challenge, bullying, or a lack of self-confidence, once you get over the first challenge, there will be another one, and you will be stronger because of the first, and then the second challenge will make you stronger once you have got passed that and onto the third. You do get to choose who you wish to be, and you get to choose whether you allow others to stop you.

You are gorgeous sister, and you get to create any kind of stage you want for yourself and your life.

So go for it, and if you need a sister to cheer you on, reach out! Reach out to me, or any of the ladies here in this book. Reach out to those in your community taking part in the activities you wish to take part in because you will find your tribe, and your tribe will love you.

Keep believing in you,
With love gorgeous,
Annie xox.

REFLECTIONS

REFLECTIONS

REFLECTIONS

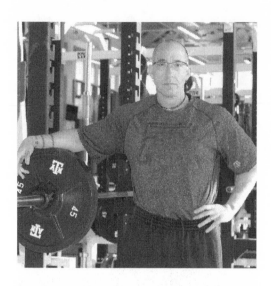

RAYCHELLE ELLSWORTH
UNITED STATES

Raychelle Ellsworth is one of the most highly regarded strength and conditioning coaches in the United States. In 2007, the Texas A&M volleyball strength and conditioning coach received the most prestigious honor awarded in her profession by being named Master Strength and Conditioning Coach by the Collegiate Strength and Conditioning Coaches association (CSCCa). At the time, she was one of only 60 in the country to hold the esteemed honor, and she remains one of only a few select females to have earned the distinction.

After completing her collegiate volleyball career at Texas A&M, she was promoted to Restricted Earnings coach. Her first full-time collegiate coaching gig was at the University of Washington in 1995–96. She returned to her alma mater in '96 and now serves as the Director of Sports Performance as well as a professor of practice in the A&M kinesiology department master's exercise physiology program.

Throughout her 20-plus years with the A&M athletic department, Ellsworth has earned tremendous respect from the A&M coaches, as well as the student-athletes, and she was recognized for her leadership, dedication, and inspiration by being voted the 1999–2000 Texas A&M Coach of the Year by the student-athletes. With the award, Ellsworth became the first non-head coach and first support staff member to receive the honor.

CHAPTER SIX
DARE TO BE GREAT

Our past shapes us, it does NOT define us. I was raised in a small town in Texas and raised on a small ranch. It was a great way to grow up, and I learned some life lessons along the way. Some of these were to do things right the first time or you would be repeating the job. That there were no specific "women's" jobs and "men's" jobs, there were just jobs. I was expected to hammer on fences, mow the lawn, drive the tractor, work cattle, haul hay, and feed the cattle. The biggest lesson I learned was that no one was coming to save me… you just find a way to get the job done, period. No excuses.

I spent many summer days on the tractor thinking. Marveling at the toughness of both my mother and father as they both worked full-time jobs and then came home to work more every day on the ranch and for other ranchers doing hay work. Days started for both of them early in the morning and lasted until the sun set and we could no longer see well enough to keep cutting, racking, baling, or hauling hay. I envied my schoolmates who would spend the day hanging out or going to the pool to waste away the days. My days were spent hot and dusty, trying to adjust the umbrella that provided a bit of relief from the brutal Texas sun. I very slowly came to the resolution that I didn't want to do this the rest of my life. But what did I want to do?

I am really competitive, and so when my parents allowed me to start playing sports at school starting in the 7th grade, I was super excited. Some may take this opportunity for granted, but both of my parents were denied this by their parents because it was such a hardship as both lived in the country and were needed at home to help with chores. I quickly excelled for my teams, mainly because I was stronger than any of the other girls and had the mental toughness between my ears. Both primarily due to growing up in the environment I did. The summer between my 8th grade year and the start of high school, I met someone who would end up changing my life. He was the newly hired coach for all of the girls' sports at the high school. I still remember the first conversation I had with Coach Larry Tidwell. I was walking through the gym and he asked me if I could touch the net hanging from the basketball rim. I smiled and I ran and jumped up and slapped the backboard that was quite a bit higher than the net. He asked me my name, what my parents did, and if I was interested in playing for him. I beamed.

I was so excited to tell my parents what happened that day. I could not wait for the summertime to be over and to show up to 2-a-days for volleyball. I was nervous and excited. All of the girls that would be playing volleyball reported, and we started doing drills. I was nervous because freshmen through seniors would all be evaluated and then divided up into two teams, junior varsity and varsity. Every day, twice a day we came to the unairconditioned gym and sweated, sweated, SWEATED! I vividly remember going to the locker room to wring out my practice shirt and then putting it back on to continue practice. It was hard, but I loved every minute of it. Coach Tidwell was fair but demanding, and all I wanted to do was prove to him that I was worthy to put on that uniform. By the start of school, I was thrilled to find out I made the varsity team. In fact, I made the varsity team in every sport I played as a freshman. I wasn't the most skilled, but I was certainly very physical, athletic, and worked hard.

I can't remember when Coach Tidwell told me, but at one point he said he thought I was talented enough to get a college scholarship. I had no frame of reference of what that truly meant at the time, but I was excited nevertheless. I worked my butt off during the school year, and in the summers, I was back on the tractor, with my parents always allowing me leave to go and practice and play in summer leagues. By my junior year, I was starting to get recruiting letters, so I knew I had a chance to see Coach Tidwell's dream for me become reality. Now, the reality of the situation is that Texas is a huge state. And there are tons of amazing athletes that get overlooked every year. So when I had a chance to go on some recruiting trips and be offered a scholarship, I felt enormous pride, and truth be told, stress. I finally picked my choice and signed my letter of intent to play volleyball at Texas A&M University. This is one of the biggest universities in the country.

All throughout high school I had been free of major injuries. Once I signed with Texas A&M as a senior, things changed. My soon to be college coach told me I needed to start playing volleyball in the spring with a club team. Club volleyball was not anywhere as popular and pervasive as it is now. I had to drive to Houston (100 miles away) a couple of times a week to practice and compete on the weekends. It was during one of these practices I hurt my knee. I ended up having knee surgery and walking down the aisle to accept my high school diploma on crutches. I spent six weeks in an immobilizer, and although I couldn't play any sports, my parents still found a way for me to rake hay all summer on the tractor, immobilized or not. Needless to say, I could not wait to get to college!

When I reported to A&M, I was technically released from my injury to start full activity, however within two weeks of practice I reinjured the same knee with the same injury and I was headed back to surgery and rehab. I was devastated because I wanted to play so badly, but in hindsight, it was a blessing because although I was very athletic, I was totally outclassed from a volleyball skill set point of view. All of my teammates had had several years of year-round volleyball practice under their belts since they played club volleyball, and thus their skill level was amazing. I on the other hand played four seasons of high school volleyball and a shortened club season. I needed the extra year to try to catch up from a skill point of view. My favorite place on campus was called the Netum Steed weight room. This is where all the athletes trained to get stronger, more explosive, and hopefully more resistant to injury. It was breathtaking. It had big glass windows, turf on the floor, and lifting equipment from end to end, and it was right next to Kyle Field, the home of the Fighting Texas Aggie football team. Whenever the volleyball team went there to train, I was giddy. I loved training and I love muscles! I can tell you the first time I fell in love with a super muscular body. It was 1977 and "The Incredible Hulk" was debuting. Lou Ferrigno was a bodybuilder who had been cast to play the "hulk." I remember staring at the screen at this huge man, painted green and wearing these pants that didn't fit right, and him flexing. All I could think of is "I want to look like that." Now I realize that probably most 8-year-old girls don't think like that, but I was hooked. I think that was the beginning of me wanting to always be strong. Growing up, I did all the things boys did, especially on the farm, so in my mind, wanting to look as muscular and be as strong as possible seemed natural.

So, I was redshirted. That is what they call an athlete that gets an extra year of eligibility due to a season-ending injury. But that redshirt year was hard, really hard. I didn't get to travel with the team, and I spent time at rehab while my teammates were practicing, getting better and better. Every time I went home to my small town, everyone would be asking why I wasn't playing. I felt ashamed that I had gotten hurt again. When an athlete from such a small town gets a scholarship to a major university, it is a very big deal. And so, when I couldn't play that first year, I felt like I was letting so many people down, including Coach Tidwell. I was also in for a big culture shock. I came from such a small town that we only had three stop lights and wasn't even big enough for a Walmart. Now I'm in a college town with multiple lanes going each direction and a mall! Some of my classes were so big that there were more people in the class than in my ENTIRE high school. College was different than I expected. I had to take classes I had zero interest in. I still had no idea what I wanted to do. So after some reflection, I decided that I would do what I enjoyed… being in the gym. I decided to become a high school coach and teacher.

The next year, I was eligible to play and I was having a blast. I earned some playing time and stepped out on the court for the first time under the lights in my uniform. I felt like it was my time all over again. I truly felt like I was part of the team and "earning my scholarship." I even managed to set a school record that I still share a part of today. Sadly, that euphoria was short lived. After a fun and successful first year and at the start of that off-season, I managed to tear my quad muscle seriously enough that I was on limited activity for another six weeks. I was so frustrated because as I mentioned before, my athleticism was off the charts but my actual volleyball skill set sucked. And again, I was missing an off-season to get better because I was restricted to walking while everyone was in the practice gym getting better and better. I was falling further and further behind. I was super frustrated and it didn't get any better. Throughout my five years of eligibility, I saw my most significant playing time that very first season after my redshirt year. After that I got caught in a vicious cycle of rehabbing, fighting my way back into playing shape and onto the court only to sustain one physical set back after another. For someone who had never missed a practice or game in high school due to injury, this was maddening. I ended up having five knee surgeries, a torn quad, and a bulging disks issue in my back that made it virtually impossible to maintain consistency in the practice gym and regain any hope of significant playing time. The only thing consistent for me was the weight room.

The weight room was my safe place. I lifted as hard as I could with whatever restrictions I had on me at the time. I think my teammates respected that. They knew realistically that I wasn't a threat to get back into the starting rotation and yet still I busted my butt in the weight room. I guess I felt like it was the right thing to do, to try to add value to the team in any way possible, to justify my scholarship. Someone once said that "an athlete dies twice, and the first death is the hardest." Truer words have never been spoken. Anyone who has identified themself as an athlete knows exactly what I'm talking about. I'm not sure mine was an easy death. I kept thinking if I can just rehab better, this will be the last time through this process and I will make my way back on the court, but that dream was quickly revealed to be just that, a dream.

With every new injury, every trip to the operating room, every trip to rehab, I felt like I was dying a slow, relentless death.

It was during the last year of my eligibility, I was walking alone from the weight room and the second coach who impacted me and changed my life approached me and asked a simple question, "what do you want to do when you graduate?" Coach Mike Clark was the head strength coach and the director of the strength and conditioning program for Texas A&M Athletics. I told him that I wanted to be a high school coach. He asked me if I ever thought of becoming a collegiate strength coach. I said "No." He asked me why not? Honestly, I had no answer. Maybe it was because we never had a full-time female strength coach on staff but all I knew was this is what I had been searching for. He asked me if I was interested in helping out when my career was over. I jumped at the chance. This was marrying the things I love... competitive athletics with my love of training in the weight room.

I worked in the weight room as soon as my final volleyball season was over until I graduated. Most of the work was "grunt" work. I cleaned the weight room, made sure everything was put back in order before closing, ran errands, and observed. Slowly, I was given small coaching duties to handle, and I must have done something right because when I graduated, I was offered the position of coaching assistant. This was a part-time job with full-time responsibilities and hours. I had a few smaller teams and helped out coaching the football groups. The football players were respectful, but I felt they didn't really think I knew much. You can't force anyone to respect you, you have to earn it. So that's what I set out to do. I thought if I train my butt off and I can get bigger, then they will trust me enough to handle spotting them and giving them lift outs. This was how I was going to get my foot in the door, so to speak, to get them to start trusting me little by little, bit by bit.

I threw myself into training. I found a training partner with bodybuilding experience and together we worked, sweated, and strained, day after day, week after week. I have always worked hard, but this was a whole different level. Training to near failure for 12–15 sets per body part is BRUTAL... but it WORKED! I got bigger and the funny thing is the more the football players saw me train and the bigger I got, the "smarter" I got in their eyes. They began not only asking for spots or handouts, but advice. I was thrilled because I made the leap from "female coach I have to respect" to "a coach who knows their shit." My confidence also started growing as well.

At the end of that year, our whole staff went to the National Strength and Conditioning Association's national conference to continue our education, network, and for me personally to take their CSCS certification exam so that I would be certified to coach at the collegiate level. While out there, I was asked to interview for a job at the University of Washington. I was flattered, but I really thought I wasn't ready to be a full-time coach yet and was loving my experience at A&M. I interviewed and literally two weeks later I was coaching at UW. This was also a culture shock for me, not only from city to city but from a work perspective as well. A&M is located in Bryan/College Station, a relatively small conservative city that is 100% a college town. Seattle on the other hand is a big, more liberal city that happens to have a major university there. I loved it, there was so much to see and do. The job was a big job. I had seven teams plus major football duties. I learned to be very organized and how to multitask very quickly.

The best part of my job ended up being sharing an office with Coach Bill Gillespie. Bill is a mountain of a man, amazingly strong and humble. Quite simply an amazing coach. I always laugh and say that my only regret taking that job was that I was so young and dumb that I didn't even know the right questions to ask Bill to take advantage of all his knowledge. We hit it off great and we became training partners. He is a lifetime drug-free powerlifting champion. I was so lucky to get to train with him and pick his brain. Many people may disregard powerlifting as having nothing to do with the athletic training preparation you do with an athlete, but they are wrong. Almost every sport has a power component to it. Power is simply Strength x Speed in a nutshell. Who better to know how to optimally drive strength levels up than people who compete in powerlifting. You just have to be smart and take concepts and apply them correctly to your training and your athletes will flourish. Bill introduced me to a lot of training ideas that I had never been exposed to. While I am so thankful for Coach Tidwell for getting me to college and Coach Clark for extending the best invitation of my life, it is Coach Gillespie who challenged me by training me with different methodologies and truly impacted my coaching philosophy choices.

I returned to my alma mater the following year when Texas A&M created a full-time position for me. It was during this time that I reflected on my college career and was disappointed that I was not to be a starter, or even play much of a significant role in those teams because of my injuries. Even though it had been years ago, I was still feeling bad about my experience. Why? I think it was because I was Ray the athlete for so long. That was my entire identity and I failed to live up to my expectations and felt like a failure and that I had disappointed my family and my town. I realized that I had been a big fish in a very small pond and had never really been challenged in high school. I was always good enough to play, to start, to have the all-district, all-regional, all-state recognitions. I think I thought if you wanted something bad enough and worked hard enough, you should be able to do whatever your goal is. I realized a lot of athletes go through something similar as I did. Moving from a small pond to a big pond is a big change, especially on a stage as big as they are stepping into in the biggest athletic conferences in America. In the Power Five conferences, there is a lot more revenue to spend because these schools within the most powerful conferences generate the most money due to their high-profile nature and television revenues. With this increased revenue comes the increased pressure to put out highly successful teams. Maybe they don't have the same struggles with injuries, but there are a lot of things that go into a sport coaches decision making to figure out who starts, who is a key reserve, and who becomes an afterthought.

That is why I decided right then and there that every athlete is important, regardless of playing time. I have created an environment in my weight rooms where my athletes respect me and how I run my program because everyone is held to the same high standards. I don't care if you are an All-American, you will do it right or you will be called out and expected to do it correctly. Too many times the stars are allowed to let things slide in practice, games, or just handling their day to day responsibilities of being on a team. They get preferential treatment. Not in my weight room. Everyone's the same. What this does is bring value to everyone that does their job. What do I value? I value things that everyone controls and don't require talent.

If you Google "10 things that require zero talent," this is what you get:

Being on time—nothing is more disrespectful than being late. You are nonverbally saying that your time is more valuable than mine or your teammates.

Work ethic—you control how you complete your task. That little voice that speaks up when things get hard or uncomfortable. "you did it good enough," "no one will know you skipped a rep." You have the power to tell that voice to shut up and to pay attention to the details that ensure you not only do the job, but do it right.

Effort—effort needs to be consistent and it needs to be present because of your intrinsic motivation. It is not my job to be your cheerleader. I always recognize effort either publicly at the end of a workout, or in private via text or conversation, but YOU need to bring it and not wait for me to drag it out of you.

Body language—this is the one element that SCREAMS at coaches and teammates alike. I watch and see who feels sorry for themselves when the conditioning gets hard. I see and appreciate the ones who are hurting but stand up and go encourage others that are struggling.

Energy—it is contagious. Everything is easier when the energy level is right. You need to set your energy/mood before you step through the door.

Attitude—remember you are here because you were chosen. You are good enough. Never doubt that.

Passion—if you don't love it, leave it.

Being coachable—be patient with yourself. New things don't always "click" right away. Keep trying. Do not make coaches repeat the same things to you every day. Learn, retain, grow.

Doing extra—everyone at this level goes to practice, watches film, eats in the dining hall, gets treatments... that is the MINIMUM. If you want to MAXIMIZE your experience, you better be willing to put in extra work that is MEANINGFUL. Work on things that you need to get better at, not the things that you like to do.

Being prepared—don't leave home without a filled water bottle and breakfast. Learn great time management skills. Listen, learn, and retain.

Funny thing is, all of these things listed above are applicable in many areas of your life including work and personal relationships. And again, they do not require talent, they just require a decision on your part to be the best version of you.

So what holds people back from truly embracing these things that require no talent?

I believe that it is a fear of failure. What if you give it everything you have and it still isn't enough? That is a very scary thought, and some people would rather hold something back so that if they don't meet their goals they have an excuse. I would say, it doesn't matter if you don't reach your goals. Working hard and putting your heart and soul into an endeavor in and of itself is something worthy and beautiful. Worst case scenario is you don't meet your goal, but I guarantee that you will be a better version of yourself than if you never committed 100% to that goal and tried. So I would challenge you to Dare To Be Great. Set a goal, develop a plan to reach that goal, commit to the ten things listed above that require no talent, and see what happens. I bet you learn a lot along the journey and it will be a worthwhile outcome.

I would like to encourage you to use the weight room as a place to set some goals regardless of your familiarity with weight lifting. As I discussed earlier, the weight room holds a special place in my heart. I feel like it truly helped save me from myself during my college playing days when I was feeling pretty worthless. It has transformed my body and has been that safe space for me to work out anger, frustration, sadness, hopelessness, and anxiety. I know it can do the same for you.

Some amazing things about the weight room or resistance training are:

1. It is a place to test yourself: 100 pounds is always 100 pounds. You have to bring your "A" game if you want to improve. This is not a place where checking the box regardless of how consistent you are will result in improvement.

2. There are no age restrictions: you can start at any point and see benefits of weight lifting. I am inspired to see women in their 60s, 70s, and even 80s kicking ass in the weight room. I guarantee you their quality of life is better than their peers who do not train. Weight lifting can increase bone density, improve balance, increase muscle mass, and can help keep body fat lower and make daily tasks easier.

3. You don't need to be athletic: find a good coach and learn the basics. Fundamentals will go a long way. Ignorance of not knowing how to lift should not be the reason you don't train.

4. Mental health is enhanced—the weight room is a great, safe place to blow off steam, help relieve stress, and increase your confidence and self-esteem.

5. Improve athletic performance: A stronger athlete typically has a more power potential. This can translate to running faster, jumping higher, changing direction more efficiently, and decreasing risk of injury.

So, no matter where you are in life's journey, whether you are an athlete, a weekend warrior, or "just plain old" you, remember **Our past shapes us, it does NOT define us.** If you don't like where you are, decide to become a better version of yourself. Sit down and write some goals. You should have a SPECIFIC bigger goal, with some smaller specific goals that will lead you to the path of the bigger goal. Make sure they are realistic. Post your goals somewhere you will see them every day. You may want to find someone to share your goal with. They can help encourage you or better yet become an accountability partner. You are worthy of EVERYTHING. Believe in yourself. **Dare to be GREAT!**

#DareToBeGreat

REFLECTIONS

REFLECTIONS

REFLECTIONS

BONUS EXERCISE

I wrote a eulogy about myself because I was questioning... What do I want to be known for?

Instead of thinking of this as a morbid exercise, think of it as a celebration of who you are.

MY EULOGY:

Here lies Laarni. The world has lost a colorful firecracker. A woman that had enough energy for a million universes. She had a smile and a belly laugh that drew you in to laugh with her. She had a strong, confident, magnetic energy that attracted people to her. She was not afraid of her truth.

She had a determined strength that showed in her training as a powerlifter and as a woman of service. She knew she wanted more for herself and she felt everyone should have a chance to be more than the constraints put upon them and live their most powerful life. Thus, she founded the Strong and Mighty Company so she could encourage and impact people to come out of the shadows.

As a women's strength advocate, she gathered and connected women's voices to build their confidence and positivity. Her nonprofit initiative the Women's Strength Initiative educates women and girls on strength, sports, and fitness.

She wanted to be strong so she could help carry and support as many people as she could. She didn't want to leave anyone behind in struggle. She leaves behind many touched lives.

If you were to write your best life, what would it say? What do you want to be known for?

Use the next pages to write your eulogy.

BONUS EXERCISE:
MY EULOGY

MY EULOGY

MY EULOGY

ABOUT THE AUTHOR

Laarni Mulvey lives in Chicago with her husband Chris and their two dogs Duke and Bruno. She loves food and cooking, trying out new recipes, as well as spending time in her garden in the summer. Gardening is a challenge every year to see how much produce she can grow as she believes homegrown veggies are not only better for you but always taste the best. Besides gardening and cooking, her additional joys include geocaching, frisbee golf, and going to get ice cream with her husband. You can find her walking around barefoot or in flip flops or hearing her distinct belly laugh somewhere. She enjoys her morning coffee so much that an idea was formed called *Let's Talk Javahhh*. It started off as a virtual coffee conversation with friends that ended up being a coffee exchange and eventually became a show. She continues to challenge her physical ability by training in powerlifting. As she says, she wants to get "SWOLE." In gym terms, get stronger. Own her space with her strength.

If you have purchased a copy of this book, we would love for you to send us a selfie of you and the book on your preferred platform:

facebook.com/RealDawnBates
instagram.com/realdawnbates
twitter.com/realdawnbates
linkedin.com/in/dawnbates

…so we can thank you in person.

With love and gratitude,
From all at Dawn Publishing

36694525R00095